THE
SPIRITUAL
MYSTERIES
OF
BLOOD

THE
SPIRITUAL
MYSTERIES
OF
BLOOD

*Its Power to Transform
Body, Mind, and Spirit*

C HRISTOPHER V ASEY, N.D.

Healing Arts Press
Rochester, Vermont • Toronto, Canada

Healing Arts Press
One Park Street
Rochester, Vermont 05767
www.HealingArtsPress.com

Healing Arts Press is a division of Inner Traditions International

Originally published in German under the title *Das Blut-Geheimnis: Ernährung und geistige Entwicklung* by Stiftung Gralsbotschaft in Stuttgart, Germany
First English edition published in 2010 under the title *The Secret of the Blood: Implications for Body, Mind, and Spirit*
Revised and expanded 2nd English edition published in 2015 by Healing Arts Press

Note to the reader: *This book is intended as an informational guide. The remedies, approaches, and techniques described herein are meant to supplement, and not to be a substitute for, professional medical care or treatment. They should not be used to treat a serious ailment without prior consultation with a qualified health care professional.*

Library of Congress Cataloging-in-Publication Data
Vasey, Christopher.
[Blut-Geheimnis. English]
The spiritual mysteries of blood : its power to transform body, mind, and spirit / Christopher Vasey, N.D. — Revised and expanded 2nd English edition.
pages cm
Originally published in German under the title: Das Blut-Geheimnis: Ernährung und geistige Entwicklung. Stuttgart : Verlag der Stiftung Gralsbotschaft, 1993.
"First English edition published in 2010 under the title: The Secret of the Blood: Implications for Body, Mind, and Spirit"—Preliminaries.
Summary: "Reveals how our blood acts as the bridge between body and spirit"— Provided by publisher.
Includes bibliographical references and index.
ISBN 978-1-62055-417-3 (paperback) — ISBN 978-1-62055-418-0 (e-book)
1. Blood. 2. Mind and body. 3. Grail movement (Bernhardt) I. Title.
QP91.V3513 2015
612.1'1—dc23
                                                    2014040405

Printed and bound in the United States by Versa Press, Inc.

10 9 8 7 6 5 4 3 2 1

Text design by Priscilla Baker and layout by Virginia Scott Bowman
This book was typeset in Garamond Premier Pro and Gill Sans MT Pro with Granjon LT Std used as the display typeface

To send correspondence to the author of this book, mail a first-class letter to the author c/o Inner Traditions • Bear & Company, One Park Street, Rochester, VT 05767, and we will forward the communication, or contact the author directly at **www.christophervasey.ch**.

Contents

The Secret of
the Blood

*I wish to fill the gaps which have so far always
remained unanswered in the souls of men as
burning questions, and which never leave any
serious thinker in peace, if he honestly seeks the
Truth.*

ABD-RU-SHIN, *IN THE LIGHT OF TRUTH:*
THE GRAIL MESSAGE

The book you are now holding in your hands, *The Spiritual
Mysteries of Blood,* is different from the other books I have
published with Healing Arts Press. Those books are mainly
concerned with physical health from a naturopathic perspective; they deal with the practical matters of detoxification and
rejuvenation, diet and the cellular terrain, and they suggest
remedies. This book is a major departure in that it is concerned

primarily with a metaphysical idea—specifically, it speaks of the immaterial spirit of the human being and the way that this spirit is connected to the body through the blood. You may ask what is the relationship between this subject and my work as a naturopath? In my practice I have often been confronted by things I have been unable to comprehend and that I later realized had a spiritual explanation. Patients came for treatment of very physical problems like rheumatism or eczema. They followed the diet I recommended; they took herbs, detoxed their bodies, and addressed all their physiological deficiencies. Such a protocol not only healed them of their physical ills, it also helped them overcome mental problems like anxiety, depression, lack of self-confidence, and various fears. How could these physical treatments have such a profound effect on the mind as well?

The most common explanation is that these kinds of naturopathic treatments work directly on the brain; to wit, as toxins are gradually eliminated, the brain receives more oxygen and thus absorbs more nutrients. But I found this explanation unsatisfying, mainly due to my conviction that our mental faculties do not originate in the brain, but rather in the human spirit. The question therefore remained open for me: How does a physical substance such as a food or an herb affect the immaterial spirit of the human being?

I felt that a piece of the puzzle was missing, and I found it one day when reading a spiritual work titled *In the Light of Truth: The Grail Message,* written between 1923 and 1937 by Oskar Ernst Bernhardt, a German better known under his pen name of Abd-ru-shin. Abd-ru-shin himself didn't form or formally support any of the spiritualist organizations that proliferated in the late nineteenth and early twentieth centuries nor was he known ever to have been a member of one; on the contrary his work seems to place a high value on individual responsibility and self-discovery—something that very much appealed to me.

Oskar Ernst Bernhardt was born on April 18, 1875, in Bischofswerda, Germany. Educated and trained as a businessman, his travels took him throughout Europe, Asia, and North America, bringing him into direct contact with peoples of many classes and cultures. He became a prolific writer of travel books, stories, and plays.

After residing for a time in New York, he moved to London in 1913. While there, the outbreak of World War I took him unawares, and because he was German he was interned on the Isle of Man for the duration of the war. His imprisonment and the seclusion it afforded him brought with it an inner deepening. At the end of the war, Bernhardt returned to Germany, fully conscious of his life's purpose: to open the path for humankind to a new knowledge of Creation, irrespective of nationality, race, creed, or any of the other means by which humanity divides itself.

Beginning in 1923, as Abd-ru-shin, a name of Persian-Arabian origin translated as "son," "workman," or "servant of the light," Bernhardt started writing spiritually themed lectures from his home in the Austrian Alps. But his prolific writing activities were cut short when the Nazis came to power in 1938. On the very day they came to power, the Nazis, threatened by Abd-ru-shin's message of human freedom and the description of a path to happiness that is attainable by anyone, arrested and imprisoned him. During his incarceration and later under house arrest, he used his solitary time to edit and arrange his 168 lectures into the present form of *The Grail Message,* though he was forbidden from publicizing his writings or making contact with his readers and was under constant surveillance by the Gestapo. Unable to continue his writing, he died in 1941.

In the Light of Truth: The Grail Message gives an explanation of the world and offers a complete survey of everything that exists between the Creator and us human beings. It has been translated into seventeen languages and is available in ninety countries worldwide and can be found online as well (www.grail-message.com).

The book states that God created human spirits and sent them in search of self-consciousness and maturity. They wandered into gross matter and acquired physical bodies in which to function on Earth. All are to learn to live by the original "Laws of Creation," which provide each human spirit with support on his earthly journey so that we can eventually return to our place of origin as mature, self-conscious entities. The book describes the mythical Holy Grail as representing a reality, the connecting point between the Creator and Creation. It provides clear answers to the fundamental questions of human existence: where the human spirit comes from, its purpose here on Earth, and where it goes after death. The book discusses fate and karma, divine justice, free will, and the mission of Jesus. On this latter subject, Abd-ru-shin says that modern human beings have become so overintellectualized that the simple, childlike belief that Jesus demanded in his time no longer suffices as a means for human beings to follow their way to God. For this reason *The Grail Message* explains Christ's teachings in a language adapted to our present way of thinking, which allows us to cultivate a certainty of conviction.

The Grail Message also touches on the question of the constitution of the human being, to wit, not only is a spirit incarnated in a body, but—and this is what struck me in particular and is the premise behind this book—is maintained in that body thanks to the blood.* In this model blood's role is not restricted to simply irrigating organic tissue, as taught in physiology. In reality it plays a much higher role—that of keeping body and spirit together. One consequence of the role blood plays as a liaison element is that any change of blood composition has repercussions on the quality of that liaison and, because of that, on the way exterior reality is perceived and felt. Our moods are thus extremely dependent on the composition of our blood.

This idea immediately captured my imagination and is the premise behind this book. This knowledge not only explains why naturopathic treatments targeting a physical problem can also influence the mind, it suggests specific tools for working on the mind in a positive way, through the blood. In fact, by altering our blood composition, we can take positive steps toward achieving mental balance and inner harmony. My hope is that this approach will open new therapeutic horizons and offer new and possibly better avenues toward self-understanding.

---

*In the appendix to this book, you will find the chapter from *The Grail Message* that speaks of the blood's true role as the bridge between the body and the human spirit.

ONE

⌖

Why Do We Eat?

Man shall give to the healthy *body what it needs.*
He shall observe it with all the care requisite
for the proper activity of this most necessary
implement in the World of Gross matter.

ABD-RU-SHIN, *IN THE LIGHT OF TRUTH:*
THE GRAIL MESSAGE

We begin our exploration with a seemingly simple question: *Why do we eat?* The answer seems obvious: we eat because our body needs food in order to function. More precisely it needs fuel (carbohydrates and fats) to provide energy to power physical activity and maintain body temperature, as well as the materials (minerals and proteins) that serve to build and maintain the body, to support growth, and to repair the wear and tear on the body's tissues. Everyone knows that we cannot avoid eating for long. The body does not contain all the fuel it needs over the course of its life. External supply is therefore indispensable. In the opinion of some, eating nothing, or fasting, would lead to death in a few days. Although this is not exactly true—it would take several weeks or even months for death to occur by starvation—it remains no less true that feeding the body is a vital necessity. We eat so that our body can survive and function.

But is that the only reason? By examining the many different ways in which people consume food, all the various modern diets that seem so different from traditional ways of eating, we can easily recognize that we also eat for many reasons other than mere nourishment.

Eating food can, for instance, have a therapeutic purpose. "Let food be your only medicine," counseled Hippocrates, the father of Western medicine. In fact, many foods are commonly used for their curative value, such as spinach and eggs for anemia, rice for high blood pressure and kidney problems, prunes in the case of constipation, milk products to avoid calcium deficiency, or potato juice for gastritis and stomach ulcers.

Diet also occupies an important place in maintaining wellness and preventing illness. A high fiber diet, for example, is needed to prevent constipation; a low-fat diet combats cardiovascular problems; foods rich in calcium are used for growth; and so on. Not only do the foods chosen for these special diets nourish the body, they have, at the same time, a therapeutic effect because they support, relieve, or reinforce the work of the different organs.

Conversely, a number of illnesses can be made worse through inappropriate food choices. For instance, diabetes is aggravated by the overconsumption of sugar, and liver problems are associated with eating excessive amounts of fat. Other diseases can be directly caused by incorrect nutrition, for example, arteriosclerosis by high consumption of cholesterol from a high-fat diet, rheumatism by too much acidic food, and immune deficiencies by inadequate intake of vitamins. And so by carefully choosing one's food, that is, by reducing or completely eliminating those foods that cause problems or by adding those that the body needs to heal or function optimally, it is possible to achieve effective disease prevention through diet alone.

In addition, food can be used to achieve certain aesthetic goals, for example, to give the body a certain shape or size considered to be more ideal by the person following the diet in question. One can barely keep track of the countless diets for losing weight, for gaining weight, for building muscle, for reducing stomach fat, and so on.

Finally, taking nourishment is accompanied quite naturally by the sensation of pleasure in eating. However, this pleasure can be pursued to excess, by overindulging and cultivating it so that it becomes a propensity. Whereas most people in the world eat to live, some people end up just living to eat. The initially healthy pleasure that accompanies the act of eating turns into a craving for food and later into gluttony, the overconsumption of food. At this point food is no longer used simply to nourish the body, but to satisfy an addiction.

The Spiritual Goals of Eating

Food is not always used just in the physical sense, as in the examples we have just described. It can also have a spiritual purpose. In this case the goal of a specific diet is not so much to achieve a certain effect on the body and its function, but rather to effect a change to the spirit. Historically, this primarily involves restrictive types of diets, diets in which one or more types of food are omitted. It is even common to see the elimination of all food for short or longer periods, that is, a time of complete fasting.

The great monotheistic religions advocate various degrees of abstinence in order to reach a spiritual goal. Christians have the period of Lent, forty-six days of fasting and abstinence starting on Ash Wednesday until Easter Sunday. Ramadan is the month during which Muslims are obliged to fast between sunrise and sunset. In the fall of each year, Jews celebrate Yom Kippur, the Feast of Atonement, and fast for twenty-four hours on this day.

In ancient times fasting for religious reasons was practiced by the Phoenicians, Assyrians, Greeks, and Romans. In Egypt participants in the ceremonies of Isis and Osiris prepared themselves by a period of fasting, which could last from seven to forty-two days. In Greece participants in the ceremonies of Eleusis fasted for seven to nine days.

What is the reasoning behind these periods of abstinence? What were the spiritual goals that people hoped to achieve? Because of the restrictive nature of fasting, we tend to associate it with the concept of punishment and penance, meant to help the spirit to expiate or atone for its "sins" and thereby free itself from the weight of its errors. However, in the field of health care, it is well known that fasting and highly restrictive diets actually have a cleansing and health-enhancing effect. At the physical level, this means cleansing works in the following way: when the body no longer receives the nutrients it requires from the exterior, it takes them from its own tissues through a biological process called *autolysis*. Autolysis is the internal process of breaking down body tissue and is carried out by enzymes secreted by the body itself. Autolysis literally means *self* (auto) and *digestion* (lysis).

Fortunately, the wisdom that governs all natural processes sees to it that autolysis of tissues takes place in a logical way. In effect, tissues are autolyzed in the inverse order of their usefulness. This means that it is metabolic wastes (toxins) and diseased tissues (cysts, fat deposits, tumors) that are the first to be autolyzed. As for healthy tissues and organs, these come only afterward. The heart and brain, as well as the other vital organs, are practically untouched by autolysis, even in the case of death by starvation.

Because autolysis "burns off" toxins and diseased tissues, it results in a cleansing of the body. The blood is purified and the organs are freed from wastes that may have accumulated— leading to the healing of any number of diseases caused or maintained by the accumulation of undesirable toxins.

As I have already noted, simultaneous with this purification of the body, a purification of the spirit also seems to take place. It is said that fasting and a strict diet can enhance our perception of our surroundings by affecting the sensitivity of our five senses. Those who practice fasting from one to several weeks often say that their thinking becomes clearer and that they have acquired a strength and clarity that they never experience outside of fasting. Our discernment becomes sharper and our spirit opens itself to intuitions or even sudden premonitions. Dramatic improvements or even outright curing of depression, obsessive-compulsive disorder, and mental illnesses have also been reported.

These beneficial effects on the spirit were certainly what the various religious traditions were seeking. Religious practitioners throughout the ages have recognized that the purification of the body leads to a kind of purification of the spirit, making it more receptive and more open to experiencing spiritual upliftment. By freeing oneself from the domination of the body, the desires and needs of the flesh, one can turn toward the heights, where contact with our higher powers can be established more easily. In addition to short periods of abstinence to prepare for particular ceremonies, longer-term dietary instructions have often been provided by various religions as well. It seems all religions saw a clear connection between the diet and the life of the spirit and therefore encouraged their faithful to pay attention to what they ate in order to promote the life of the spirit.

This being the case, it stands to reason that if a short period of abstinence could have a favorable effect on the spirit, then a less stringent form of diet followed over a longer time, perhaps over a whole lifetime, would provide even more beneficial spiritual effects.

That the diets recommended for spiritual practitioners exclude alcohol and other drugs that alter the physical senses and reduce self-control and discernment will not surprise anyone. But the idea of restricting or totally eliminating a common food item like meat is more complicated.

Contrary to certain primitive tribal people, who ate the eyes of their enemies slain in battle in order to see better, or their tongues to be able to speak better, or their hearts to have more courage and strength, later religions conceived of the idea that by *not* eating animal flesh, one could avoid awakening the animal forces within human beings.

Eating large amounts of meat actually increases sexual drive and acts as a stimulant in humans. A meat diet can make a person more active and excitable and even aggressive or violent. In contrast it is well known that a diet without meat greatly loosens the bond between the spirit and the body. Vegetarianism tends to reduce interest in material things in general, while physical passions are attenuated. A person who follows this kind of diet will be less interested in material possessions and will be less greedy, ambitious, and confrontational. Self-control, including mastery of desires and impulses, becomes easier. Opening toward higher values is favored on such a diet.

These effects are even more evident, but can become unhealthy, when the diet is even more restrictive and, in addition to meat, other foods are eliminated as well. This can happen with a vegan diet, where only plant-based foods (fruit, vegetables, cereals, and legumes) are allowed, or a fruit diet, where only fresh, dried, and oleaginous fruit comprise the basis of nutrition, as contrasted with a less restrictive, more moderate lacto-vegetarian diet, which still allows certain animal products such as eggs and milk. In the extreme a person who follows these kinds of highly restrictive dietary regimes might completely turn away from material things and could even lose touch with reality. Those around such a person will say that he is ungrounded or "has his head in the clouds." Such a person might even go to such an extreme that he acknowledges that the physical world no longer matters.

Food as a Means to Enhance Spiritual Development

The possibility of influencing one's spiritual and psychic development through food is such a long-standing tradition that students of the occult still regularly use this, as well as other techniques, to promote the development of special psychic abilities such as mediumship, clairvoyance, clairaudience, or visionary experiences.

Today more and more people are following nontraditional diets, initially not for spiritual goals, but as a path to good health. The dramatic changes that are then experienced on the inner plane as a result of altering one's diet eventually lead the person to realize how much food can affect the spirit. So for many it starts out as a quest for good health, which then becomes a quest for development of the total person. Under these circumstances it is not uncommon to hear people speak of the spiritual progress they have made since they changed their diet.

Yet we may well ask if this effect on the spirit is real or just an illusion, and if the followers of these restrictive diets are only deluding themselves. These questions deserve to be asked, because up until now no one has been able to explain precisely how food can have this effect on the spirit and why purification of the body can also bring about a purification of the spirit.

If the spirit were identified with the brain, this influence would be easy to explain. Good nutrition provides the brain with all the minerals and vitamins it needs, and cleansing the blood improves the circulation and therefore oxygen uptake by the brain. But in the thinking outlined above, the spirit is regarded as the *nonmaterial* principle of man, as what is commonly called his "soul." We therefore have to ask ourselves how something material like food can influence something nonmaterial like the spirit.

Even if the brain were to be considered as the location of the spirit, we are still confronted by a significant problem, in the sense that it would mean that spiritual development depends primarily on proper nutrition of the brain—on diet alone—and not on the efforts and perseverance of the person.

To understand how food affects the spirit, we must first know exactly what the spirit really is.

TWO

∽

What Is the Spirit?

Do you not clearly notice a difference between the form and your "ego"? Between the body that is subject to change and yourself, the spirit, which is eternal?

ABD-RU-SHIN, *IN THE LIGHT OF TRUTH:*
THE GRAIL MESSAGE

Today we find mainly two different points of view regarding the nature of the spirit. For some the spirit is something non-material that resides within the physical body during its life on Earth. For others it is material in nature and resides within the brain. *Resides* is not exactly the right term, because in this second point of view, the spirit and brain are not seen as being two different things, but rather one and the same thing.

This identification of the spirit with the brain is implied in certain expressions. It's often said of great thinkers, scientists, or intellectuals, that they are "men of great spirit" or that such a person is "rich in spirit" if she impresses us with a highly intelligent way of speaking. Scientific studies of the brain seemingly support this point of view.[1]

Researchers have in fact discovered that the brain is divided into different areas, or "brain centers," and that each brain center has a specific function. For example, there is a brain center for vision, one for hearing, one for moving the fingers or the legs, a brain center for writing, for reading, and so on. Sensitive electroencephalogram (EEG) instruments show us that when a person writes, only the brain center responsible for written language is activated, but no other brain center. In addition, experiments conducted with the help of minute electrodes inserted into the brain demonstrate that stimulating a specific part of the brain with a small electric current triggered a response corresponding to that brain center. For instance, in one study test subjects started to speak when the speech center was stimulated or lifted the right arm when the motor center for the right arm was stimulated.[2]

Those who advocate this second way of looking at the spirit will ask what more proof do we need in order to accept that all human attributes are based in the brain and that the brain and the spirit are one and the same, especially since we know that the destruction of any one brain center leads to a simultaneous loss of the corresponding conscious ability, as when, for example, the speech center is damaged after a stroke and the patient loses his ability to speak. And although the brain centers for the will and the personality have yet to be discovered, some scientists contend that it is only a question of time before we will finally be able to discard once and for all the "hypothesis" of the existence of a nonmaterial spirit that is distinct from the body.

This contention, however, will ultimately lead to disappointment, not only for various reasons that we shall cover later on, but also for one primary reason that science itself has already discovered. Sir John Eccles, a 1963 recipient of the Nobel Prize for Medicine for his research on the brain, writes in his book *The Self and Its Brain,* "The brain, which is a machine comprised of neurons, is absolutely incapable of carrying out the required integrations (uniting and processing all the elements that make up our human condition). For this, an active and independent spirit, which uses the brain as an instrument, is needed."[3] In other words the brain, because of its very structure, is not capable of being the center of the conscious personality and therefore cannot be synonymous with the spirit. It is simply not capable of it.

The Brain, a Tool

The brain is only a machine, albeit a highly developed machine, but all the same a machine, one that serves a higher principle that is independent and distinct from the brain's purely mechanical abilities: it serves the spirit, the true core of our personality.

To understand the abilities as well as the limitations of the brain, we can compare it to a computer, because the functions of the two are quite similar. A computer can do absolutely nothing until we supply it with data or information to work on. In computer jargon we must feed it with data. But that still does not suffice. The computer must also be programmed or instructed as to what to do with this information; after all, it is only a machine that cannot think independently. By programming it with software, we tell it what to do. Only then can the computer perform its work of assembling data, sorting, adding, subtracting, or performing other operations. The work it performs is carried out in logical sequence, step by step, mathematically relating one piece of information to another in order to obtain a result, and each new result is added in turn to the database. And so the answers that a computer can give to our questions are derived from supplied data and a program. What it can do for us therefore always depends on what we first give it, and this always has to be the same category as the information we want back from it. A computer cannot possibly produce anything totally new or of a different category than its input. It has no creative ability; it can only process the data provided to it.

Our brain works the same way. Bit by bit, little by little, through education and the experiences of daily life, our brain gathers the information that forms its "database." It is also through education and experience that the brain acquires its ability to work on this data, that is, its program.

A computer can produce impressive results, but there are a certain number of things that it just cannot do. It cannot enjoy its work, it cannot become stirred up by an idea, and it has no sense of responsibility. By itself it can never imbue its work with a sense of beauty or any of the higher values that we humans possess, such as a sense of justice or a sense of right and wrong. Nor can it become inspired or obtain a sudden intuition about how to solve a problem. It is also impossible for it to become impatient with its operator—it cannot become annoyed over the work that it is asked to do, and it cannot refuse to do it either.

Love, hate, patience, a sense of what is good and beautiful—all these are not qualities that a machine can have, but they are specific attributes of the human being, or more accurately, the human spirit. Neither can the brain, which has similar capabilities to a computer, recognize beauty, goodness, or justice. These abilities belong to the spirit. People love with their hearts, are annoyed, moved, or rebel with their whole being, not with their brain.

The Subordination of the Brain to the Spirit

If the brain and the spirit are indeed two entirely different things, and if the brain is but the tool of the spirit, it must be possible to find examples or circumstances that confirm this. For instance, how about when the tool (the brain) follows its own logic (the program), but the user (the spirit) overrides it; or how about when the user becomes involved in something without any participation from the tool, in the same way that a person who works at a computer can lead a life completely independent of her computer when she leaves work.

Examples of this can be seen in the experiment mentioned earlier, where brain centers were stimulated by microelectrodes. In this case the electrical stimulation was activated from a distance and without the knowledge of the test subject. In the experiment the researcher could induce specific reactions in the test subjects by stimulating well-defined areas of the brain. For instance, he could make the subjects lift one leg, tell a funny story, cry, feel afraid or aggressive, all according to the area of the brain stimulated. On one occasion something totally surprising happened during the course of the experiment. One of the subjects whose brain was being stimulated in a certain area became aggressive and threatening toward the researcher during the session, clenching his fists and shouting, "Fortunately for you, doctor, I don't want to hurt you, because otherwise . . ." This person found himself compelled to become violent, but he held himself back. In other words the electrical impulse triggered an aggressive reaction at the level of the brain, but there was something else within this person that helped him restrain his aggressiveness and control his brain's reaction. The brain had become subject to a superior authority: the spirit, which itself could not be affected by the electrical impulse.

Clear evidence of the fact that the spirit is distinct from the brain and is not affected by what happens to the latter can be found in cases of damage to certain areas of the brain. As is generally known, damage to any brain center brings about the loss of the corresponding physical ability. There is one report of a man who underwent total ablation of the left hemisphere of his brain. Because of the loss of function in the speech center, which is situated in that hemisphere, the man lost his ability to speak. Yet despite this, and contrary to all expectations, eight months later he was speaking normally again.[4]

The first question that arises is how could his ability to speak be restored after his speech center had been destroyed? We could also ask ourselves where the man's restored ability came from, since the "data" for it had disappeared. If the spirit and the brain are one and the same, then these kinds of questions would remain without any satisfactory answers. The permanent destruction of the speech center would make it impossible to ever restore the man's ability to speak. As the restoration was not due to a transfer of information from one part of the brain to another, how then did it happen?

But if we look at these questions in a different light and acknowledge that the brain is but a tool of the spirit, subordinate to it, then everything becomes clear. The so-called speech center located within the brain is merely a place where information about speech is stored but is not the true speech center. The actual ability to speak lies in the spirit of the person. In other words it is not the tool that thinks and speaks, but rather the user (the spirit), who, by means of its tools (the brain and speech organs), speaks.

Again, let's look at the computer metaphor: the deletion of data stored in a computer does not simultaneously delete the knowledge of the user, who can easily reenter the data and the program into the computer. In our example above, the spirit was able to re-create the speech center in another part of the brain because *the basic ability continued to exist within the spirit*. It is less a question of relearning than a transfer of information from the spirit to another part of the brain.

The Eternal Spirit

Let us now consider some examples of the spirit experiencing something without the participation of the brain. We begin with a report of an event that occurred during a patient's stay in a hospital, an out-of-body experience, which is more common than many would believe.

I was in the hospital in Sion because of a diabetic crisis.
I had received treatment and was feeling better. It was in
the morning, I no longer remember all the details. What I
do know is that I was wandering around the room, feeling
detached. I distinctly felt that I was floating. I felt light.
Suddenly I saw from above an elderly woman stretched out
on a bed, appearing to be asleep. I did not immediately recognize that it was my own body. There was a loud noise;
I don't know where it came from. I was startled, and then
I realized that I was the one lying on the sheet, dressed in
my badly stained dressing gown. I thought, *So I'm now*
supposed to get back again into this broken-down, overweight
body of a woman? But do I really have to? This was not
expressed in words but in thought. I had to reenter my
body. The time had not yet come for me to abandon it. I
carefully let myself slide inside, as if I was a cloud of vapor
that entered through the pores of the skin of this person,
who was me. After a moment I opened my eyes. I saw the
room and the sick woman in the next bed. I was lying on
my bed, in my stained dressing gown. How did this excur-
sion happen? How did I leave my body?[5]

If this person had asked herself how she was able to leave
her body, we might also ask ourselves what it was that left her
body. It was certainly not her brain. Nevertheless, the woman
was still alive and was able to experience something: She saw
her body stretched out on the bed. She heard a loud noise and
was startled by it. She then thought that she should reenter her
body, and so she slid back into it again.

Someone who would question the truthfulness of this

account or its explanation might say that it was all just an illusion. He would perhaps say that the woman only had the *impression* that she had left her body, that in reality she was just dreaming and had actually remained in her body the whole time, and that all this took place "in her head." If everything that happened was only in her head, then it would mean that she had experienced this situation with her brain, something an EEG would have been able to show. Yet there are many cases in which EEGs were taken of persons that showed no brain activity, although the individuals in question later reported having experienced situations that for them were very real and powerful.

In medicine a flat EEG and no heartbeat are sufficient evidence to pronounce a person dead. Such tests are undertaken, for example, in the emergency room of a hospital to see whether accident victims or someone seriously ill is still alive, to determine whether or not resuscitation efforts should be undertaken. If these tests show that an accident victim is no longer alive, nobody would expect that she would be able to see, move, or feel anything because, after all, she is dead, right? And yet there are shocking examples of hundreds of people who have had just such experiences of being pronounced clinically dead and then revived, as reported by the American physician Raymond Moody.[6] In his groundbreaking book, Dr. Moody cites numerous instances of people who told him what they experienced while they were dead, that is, during the short or even longer periods of time between the moment their hearts stopped beating and their brains stopped functioning, and when resuscitation attempts were successful.

These stories are undoubtedly true, because they were recounted—and experienced—by people of different ages and sexes who did not know one another, had no contact with one another, and who belonged to very different social and cultural groups. What is striking in all these accounts is that all of these people provided similar accounts of how their lives continued right after their physical deaths. But what is most remarkable—and this is the main point here—is that while these people were living the events they described, their EEGs remained flat. Their brains played no part in what happened. They were clinically dead.

For those who would think that despite this evidence the brain must still have been in some way or other connected with the events, let us consider another example, in which the experience of the spirit continued on through more than one lifetime and obviously through more than one physical body.

In every part of the world, in every country, race, ethnic, and cultural group, there are cases of children who have reported events that they claim to have experienced, but which did not take place in their current lifetime.

The following is a typical story:

A girl named Maria, who lived in a small town in Illinois, died at the age of fifteen. Three years later her mother moved to another town and gave birth to a little girl, to whom she gave the name Nellie. Nellie, however, insisted that people call her Maria, maintaining that this was her real name, the name her parents had given her.

One day, visiting for the first time the same small town in Illinois where the family had once lived, little Nellie immediately recognized the house in which her family used to live and also recognized different people, even though she had never met them, at least not in this lifetime. Nellie then gave an exact description of the school in the town and expressed the wish to go to see it. When she got there, she proceeded, without any hesitation, to her classroom and pointed out the desk where Maria had once sat.

A story of this kind could be dismissed as a product of pure imagination if the numerous reported facts, especially the details given by Nellie, could not have been checked on the spot and verified in the presence of the parents and neighbors who had surrounded the child in her previous life as Maria. The task was taken on by Ian Stevenson, a research professor of psychiatry at the University of Virginia School of Medicine, to conduct stringent and systematic examinations of more than 2,500 cases of this kind. Stevenson concluded that these reports were authentic and that they described real events experienced by the subjects in their previous lifetimes.[7]

Some people have difficulty accepting this conclusion because it is generally accepted that the memory of events is stored only in the brain. Therefore, returning to the aforementioned story, according to conventional belief everything that had been recorded in Maria's brain would have been lost with it at the time of the dissolution of her body at death. But Nellie was able to recount events from her past life as Maria, even though her present brain had played no part in experiencing these events and consequently could not have recorded these memories. The conclusion must be that Nellie's recollections were not stored in Maria's brain, but rather in something that survived Maria after her death, which was now part of Nellie. This "something" is not physical or material; it is spirit.

The Nature of Spirit

The preceding examples demonstrate that the spirit and the brain are two distinct things. As the brain is unquestionably material in nature, the spirit itself must be composed of something different, something nonmaterial. So what is the spirit, really? *In the Light of Truth: The Grail Message* describes the spirit as "the only truly living part of a human being." Abd-ru-shin continues:

> Spirit is not wit and not intellect! Nor is spirit acquired knowledge. It is erroneous, therefore, to call a person "rich in spirit" because he has studied, read, and observed much, and knows how to converse well about it, or because his brilliance expresses itself through original ideas and intellectual wit.
>
> Spirit is something entirely different. It is an independent **consistency,** coming from the world of its homogeneous species, which is different from the part to which the earth and thus the physical body belong. The spiritual world lies higher; it forms the upper and lightest part of Creation. Owing to its consistency, this spiritual part in man bears within it the task of returning to the Spiritual Realm, as soon as all the material coverings have been severed from it. The urge to do so is set free at a very definite degree of maturity, and then leads the spirit upwards to its homogeneous species, through whose power of attraction it is raised.
>
> Spirit has nothing to do with the earthly intellect; only with the quality which is described as "deep inner feeling." To be rich in spirit, therefore, is the same as "having deep inner feelings," but not the same as being highly intellectual.[8]

This definition not only states that the spirit is not part of the body (and is therefore not synonymous with the brain), it clarifies the origins of each. The spirit comes from the spiritual plane, whereas the body belongs to the earthly plane. This definition is in complete agreement with the teachings of Christ. When Christ said, "The spirit is willing, but the flesh is weak," does that not mean that since the spirit is not weak like the flesh, it must be of a different nature? In other words the spirit is not made of flesh and therefore cannot be part of the brain.

Abd-ru-shin says the spirit issues from the spiritual realm—Paradise—and can return there after a path of development that, among other events, leads it to incarnate in a physical body. Between the spiritual and earthly planes, there exist other planes of different kinds, as Christ mentions briefly when he speaks of the many dwelling places (planes) in his father's house (Creation). On its journey through the different planes to incarnate on Earth, the spirit puts on, one after another, different cloaks, or bodies, belonging to each of the different planes, the last one being the earthly body we know. The best known of these finer coverings, or bodies, is the astral body. It is the best known because its species is most closely related to our material, earthly body.

The Descent of the Spirit into the Body

The need to incarnate, that is, to enter (*in*) a body of flesh (*carne*) of the same nature as the plane into which the spirit wishes to penetrate, is logically understandable. The spirit needs this physical human body to be able to experience the plane in question; the physical body therefore serves it as a tool to enable the spirit to see, feel, and to move around. Without the physical body, the spirit would have no connection with this plane and could not therefore become active in it; the difference in species would not permit it. Thus the goal of incarnation, which is for the spirit to live through the experiences of life on Earth in order to mature, could never be achieved.

The spirit does not play a secondary role in our life; it is not just an accessory put at our disposal. The spirit is who we really are. The physical body, the astral body, and the finer bodies are only cloaks or tools used by the real *I,* which is spirit.

The Grail Message describes the spirit further:

> The spirit is everything; it is the true being, thus man himself. When, together with the other cloaks, he also wears the physical body, he is called earthman. If he lays aside his earthly cloak, he is considered by earthman to have become a soul. When he finally lays aside the finer coverings which still surround him, he remains spirit alone, this being his true nature, which he has always been.
>
> Thus the various designations are merely adapted to the species of the cloaks covering the spirit, which could not exist on their own if they were not embraced by the spirit, which glows through them.[9]

And since the physical body belongs to the plane of dense matter, the spirit therefore bears no more similarity to this body than it does to the material plane itself. How then is it possible for the spirit to incarnate in the body, take possession of it, animate it, and control it? What gives it the ability to form a bridge over the gulf created by the huge difference in composition between itself and the dense physical body?

Actually, this bridge is composed of the different bodies in which the spirit cloaks or envelopes itself during its descent through the different planes, from the spiritual plane down to the earthly plane. However, it should be noted that each different body belongs to a different plane and consequently has a different composition. The question therefore remains: How can the spirit, surrounded by its different coverings, connect with the dense physical body? The answer to this question, *The Grail Message* says, is through the blood. This is the secret of the blood.

THREE

∽

The True Purpose
of Blood

*The blood! How much swings forth from this
word, how rich and strong are all the impressions
it is able to produce, and what a never-ending
source of conjecture is contained in this one
significant word!*

ABD-RU-SHIN, *IN THE LIGHT OF TRUTH:
THE GRAIL MESSAGE*

It is generally accepted that the task of the blood is to irrigate
the tissues of the body so that the cells have a constant supply of oxygen and nutrients. We also understand its role in
the removal of metabolic wastes and that it conveys hormonal
messages from cell to cell. We know as well that blood plays
an important role in the body's immune system. According
to science the purpose of blood is to serve the body faithfully,

to always be available to support it in many ways. In order of importance, the body comes first, while the blood, although indispensable, remains subordinate and therefore comes second. But is this really the case? Is blood subordinate to the body? This question, as we shall see, goes far beyond any simple scientific or intellectual interest; it opens us to new horizons of understanding who we truly are.

The Primacy of Blood

The interdependence between the body and the blood appears to be so close that it is seemingly impossible to determine which one really comes first. However, by examining the facts, we can arrive at a definitive answer to this question.

The first hint comes from the medical procedure known as dialysis. During dialysis arterial blood passes through a specially developed filtering machine that cleanses it of waste products such as urea. The cleansed blood is then led back into the body through a vein. This means of blood cleansing is used for patients whose kidneys are too badly damaged to do it on their own. It is significant that 300 to 400 grams of urea can be filtered out during twenty-four hours of dialysis, whereas the presence of only two grams of urea per liter of blood is considered to be toxic. Since our body has only about five to seven liters of blood, one has to ask where the 300 to 400 grams of urea come from. It is obviously not contained in the blood, since the presence of only a very few grams of urea in the blood would be fatal. It turns out that the urea is taken back up by the body, or more accurately, by the tissues, and is only released into the blood during dialysis.

If the body is "sacrificed" in this way, that is, if it has to bear the toxic burden of the excess urea and thereby safeguard the normal composition of the blood, does this not mean that the blood is more important than the body? And in this case couldn't one say that the body is in service to the blood?

That blood ranks ahead of the body also becomes evident in the opposite situation, that is, when the danger threatening the normal composition of the blood does not come from an excess of a toxic substance from within, as seen in the previous example, but from a deficiency of an external substance that is needed.

Normally, blood contains a certain number of alkaline substances (calcium, sodium, magnesium, etc.) that it uses to neutralize or buffer acids that threaten its normal pH, or its degree of acidity. When the level of acid is too high and remains so, these alkaline minerals are used up and another defense mechanism comes into play, as alkaline minerals are drawn from various tissues of the body such as the bones, nails, skin, or hair follicles, in order to restore the normal pH of the blood.

This defense mechanism is important because if the pH of the blood varies too far from its ideal value, the body can no longer function properly. It becomes ill and shows signs of disturbed consciousness. If the organism needs to continually resort to this defense mechanism, there is a risk that the body can become dangerously demineralized. And if the cause of the imbalance in pH is not soon corrected, the continued extraction of alkaline minerals robs the body of minerals necessary for its health, and it suffers severe consequences: the bones decalcify and become porous, the teeth develop cavities, become brittle, and fall out, and the skin becomes dry and cracked. Here again, the primacy of the blood is clearly illustrated, in that the body literally sacrifices itself for it. To maintain the normal content of alkaline minerals in the blood, minerals are drawn from tissues and organs, even if these tissues and organs are seriously harmed in the process.

These two examples are neither unique nor unusual. The same defense mechanisms occur with waste products other than urea and with nutrients other than alkaline minerals. It is well known from the study of physiology that the body is constantly working to provide the blood with an ideal level of vitamins, minerals, amino acids, and other constituents, by absorbing them from the digestive system or, if the diet does not supply them, from the body's own tissues. The body may then become seriously ill just to save the blood.

Therefore, contrary to what is commonly believed, the blood is not secondary to the body, but rather, the body is in service to the blood, and with the help of all the resources of its organs, it stays on guard to maintain the ideal composition of the blood.

Without blood, the body can do nothing; it dies. The term *lifeblood* is defined by *Webster's* as "blood regarded as the seat of vitality; a vital or life-giving force or component." This definition contains much wisdom. This connection between blood and life itself is the reason for the many other striking expressions found in different languages having to do with the blood. As long as it is flowing through our veins, life flows within us. If a vessel bursts and blood gushes out, it is said that life itself departs, that the person's "life is flowing out" of him.

"Blood is a very special juice," said Goethe. Actually, it is a *sacred* juice. The chants and songs and rituals of traditional peoples that honor blood acknowledge that it is uppermost in importance. We encounter tales of blood in Homer's *Odyssey* (Book XI), "As soon as he had tasted the blood he knew me, and weeping bitterly stretched out his arms towards me to embrace me," as well as in the Book of Exodus, "And the blood shall be to you for a token upon the houses where ye *are:* and when I see the blood, I will pass over you, and the plague shall not be upon you to destroy *you,* when I smite the land of Egypt" (12:13). "And Moses took the blood, and sprinkled *it* on the people, and said, Behold the blood of the covenant, which the LORD hath made with you concerning all these words" (24:8). If blood was subordinate to the body, there would be more odes to the primacy of the body, not the blood.

Yet some might say that to assign primacy to the blood contradicts the science of physiology, which states that it is the body that produces the blood. This means that the secondary or subordinate body produces the primary or superior blood. How could that be possible? One might be tempted to say, as French writer Paul Valéry says, that the one is equally as important as the other: "The only work of the body is to maintain the blood . . . But blood itself has no other job than to give the body which generated it whatever it needs in order to function. The body produces the blood, which produces the body, which produces the blood."[1] But this way of looking at it does not really further our understanding and just locks us into a pointless chicken-or-egg cycle.

Blood's Relationship to Spirit

The examples provided above show what happens in extreme situations, when the organism as a whole, body and blood, is threatened: the body is sacrificed to save the integrity of the blood. It may therefore be logically concluded that the blood is the more important of the two, and the body exists to support the blood. But this leads to a fundamental question: If the body exists for the blood, then what is the purpose of the blood? If the blood really is more important than the body, then whatever the blood exists for must be even more important than the blood itself. But what exactly is that?

To answer this question, we turn once again to *The Grail Message,* whose spiritual approach to this subject provides a metaphysical (beyond the physical) overview, something that science, being restricted to the gross physical, cannot provide. The main purpose of human blood, says Abd-ru-shin, is to *"form the bridge for the activity of the spirit on earth,* i.e., in the World of Gross Matter! This sounds so simple, and yet it holds the key to *all* knowledge about the human blood."[2]

The raison d'être of the blood is therefore to serve the spirit. The blood has to be present to form the bridge for the spirit to incarnate into the physical body. Without the blood the spirit would not be able to incarnate or to remain incarnate during its sojourn on Earth. The spirit is therefore not connected directly with the body; it is more specifically connected to the blood, and only through the blood does it then connect to the body.

Given this perspective one can understand why the body works so devotedly on behalf of the blood and even sacrifices itself for it. In other words: no blood = no bridge = no life. Furthermore, if the body lives, it is not because of the blood; the body lives because of the spirit, "the only truly living part in man," says Abd-ru-shin, by means of its connection to spirit through the blood.

The Radiating Bridge

Though as we have demonstrated it is primarily a liaison to the spirit, the blood, like the body itself, is nevertheless material in nature and is therefore not of the same composition as the spirit. To build a bridge between the two realms, material and spiritual, there has to be an additional factor present, and this factor is the *radiation of the blood*. "The radiation of the blood," asserts Abd-ru-shin, "is therefore in reality the actual bridge for the activity of the soul, and then only if this blood is of a very particular *composition suitable for the soul concerned*."[3]

Let's go to the dictionary definition of *radiation*. *Webster's* says it is "the action or process of radiating; the process of emitting radiant energy in the form of waves or particles; the combined processes of emission, transmission, and absorption of radiant energy."

Like everything material, blood radiates; it sends out invisible radiation that spreads out like waves. These waves are of a different composition than the blood itself; they are ethereal or energetic in nature. Although not exactly the same, they more closely resemble the composition of the astral body, which, apart from the physical body, is the densest of the cloaks enveloping the spirit. The astral body itself also radiates, and the coarsest of these radiations emanating from it combine with the finest radiations emanating from the blood. These two radiating energies join to form a bridge for the spirit. There is not, therefore, a direct, physical, tangible connection between the astral body and the physical body, but rather a finer bond, a *radiating bridge* that connects the astral body and the blood flowing within the physical body. This bridge is similar to the force that brings two magnets together. The connection between the two magnets is not visible, but the bond is nevertheless very strong.

These radiating energies not only serve the role of connecting the spirit with the body, they are also a means of communication between the two. Information received by the five senses of the physical body is collected in the brain, and then after processing and refinement is transmitted to the spirit over the radiation bridge. In the opposite direction, the will of the spirit, that is, the kind of response it chooses to make to the information it is given, is transmitted over the same radiation bridge to the physical brain, which then concerns itself with carrying out the desired activity in the plane of gross matter.

It is important that the radiation bridge is maintained in good condition so that the two-way flow of information works well. If not, it would be like a person who cannot hear a radio program clearly because the radio is not tuned to the same wavelength or frequency as the transmitting station. The result is a confused, inaudible transmission. This may be relatively unimportant in the case of someone listening to a radio program, but it is an absolute catastrophe for communication between the spirit and the brain—in other words the communication between our deepest and true self and our everyday consciousness.

To fully experience life on Earth, our spirit absolutely needs a strong and healthy blood radiation. The blood radiation must resonate with the vibrations coming from its earthly surroundings, and at the same time it must provide a reliable mechanism through which the spirit can fully express itself and experience the world of matter. And the quality of the blood radiation, as stated in *The Grail Message,* depends absolutely on the composition of the blood. Any change in composition brings about a change in the blood radiation and thereby a change in the spirit-body connection. As long as the body works diligently to maintain an ideal blood composition, it will be able to provide the cells with a constant supply of necessary nutrients, but more importantly it will be able to maintain the radiation bridge in the best possible condition at all times.

Every bridge, of whatever kind, has at least two points of support, one on each end. It is exactly the same here. The blood radiation bridge depends on two factors or two anchor points: the radiation of the blood and the radiation emanating from the spirit.

A Short History of Blood

As the nature of any form of radiation depends on the nature of the object from which it originates (i.e., its source), it follows that every individual spirit has its own unique radiation. Indeed we are all unique, and we differ in a multitude of ways: our character traits, our qualities and our shortcomings, our abilities either latent or expressed, and so on. And just as every spirit radiates in a unique way, it needs a distinctive blood radiation that is appropriate for it and that matches the characteristics of its own radiation. But a distinctive blood radiation also implies a distinctive blood composition. It is therefore only logical that we should each have a different blood composition.

Does this information, which rests on spiritual understanding, conflict in any way with the facts? Can it be verified by the findings of physiology? To answer this question, we first have to look at the history of discoveries concerning the blood and its composition.

Knowledge about the blood was absent for a very long time. For Hippocrates, in the fourth century BCE, the veins contained nothing but air. For the second-century Greek doctor Galen, the arteries as well as the veins contained blood but it did not circulate; it had, rather, a slow reciprocating motion. One has to go forward another 1,500 years until an English doctor, William Harvey, discovered in 1623 that blood circulates and that this circulation takes place from the heart to the organs and from the organs back to the heart, which acts as a pump.

In the distant past, knowledge about the composition of blood progressed only barely. The existence of red blood cells was not discovered until the seventeenth century, and the other principal components of blood, white blood cells and platelets, was only discovered in the nineteenth century. Despite the limited knowledge of the actual composition of blood, its importance has been recognized from earliest times. But throughout the ages until relatively recently, people could only dream about replacing lost or diseased blood with new blood.

Before the first attempts at blood transfusion, patients drank fresh blood from sacrificed or slaughtered animals to try to improve or replace their own blood. At different times blood was dried and added as a powder to various foods, such as sausages, biscuits, bread, or sauces. Powdered animal blood was an ingredient in pharmaceutical products and was also used in medicinal baths. The first known attempts at blood transfusions took place in the seventeenth century. Animal blood was transfused into humans, but since animal blood is not the same as human blood, these transfusions ended in failure—the death of the patient—with the result that such practices came to a swift end.

The practice of blood transfusion resumed in the nineteenth century. This time transfusions were undertaken directly from one person's arm to another person, to avoid the problem of blood clotting, a problem that had not yet been resolved at that time. The blood of the donor flowed directly into the vein of the recipient by way of a tube connecting the two circulatory systems. Sometimes the vein of the donor was actually sewn to that of the recipient. And although human blood was used this time, numerous fatalities occurred, as one can well imagine. The blood of the donor was not always compatible with that of the recipient. Investigations into the cause of these failures led to the discovery that despite the apparent similarity in blood composition from one person to the next, everyone's blood is different and unique. The content of red cells, platelets, and so on might be the same, but the characteristics were different.

The first of these differences was discovered in the year 1900 by the Viennese doctor Karl Landsteiner. He noted four different types of red blood cells, which he divided into four groups: A, B, AB, and O. With this the modern conception of four human blood types was discovered, and the first step had been taken toward recognizing the individuality of a person's blood.

Transfusions that respected the laws of compatibility between the blood types had a high rate of success, but despite this knowledge there were deaths due to blood transfusions. The number of deaths declined, however, beginning in 1940, when Landsteiner discovered an additional property of blood, the Rhesus factor, or Rh factor, which permitted an even greater personalization of blood for transfusions. Later on, other blood groups were discovered (for instance the Kell, Duffy, and Kidd systems), leading to further decreases in the number of transfusion deaths.

The year 1952 saw a significant new step forward toward the further differentiation of blood types. The French scientist Jean Dausset discovered the existence of new markers on the membranes of white blood cells, the human leukocyte antigen, or HLA, system. Later on, other markers were discovered on blood platelets—in the serum, on the immune globulins and proteins, and even on certain enzymes of blood cells.

The more research on blood progressed, the more ways to determine the differences between the various kinds of blood entered the knowledge base. As of this writing more than thirty systems of markers have been recognized, permitting an almost infinite number of possible combinations. Still, the chances of finding a biological double are at best a billion to one.

With the current state of knowledge, science has confirmed that everyone's blood is completely unique. Its composition is always different from one person to another. This fact confirms the spiritual understanding, as revealed in *The Grail Message,* that the blood radiation is different from one person to the next because it must be distinctly appropriate to the soul in question in order to serve as a bridge for its activity.

FOUR

∽

Factors
That Influence
the Blood

*Each body creates certain definite radiations
which are absolutely essential to the spirit for its
work in the World of Matter.*

ABD-RU-SHIN, *IN THE LIGHT OF TRUTH:
THE GRAIL MESSAGE*

Since we have confirmed that the blood is the bridge
or connecting link between the spirit and the body, any
changes to the blood, be they quantitative or qualitative,
result in a change in the connection. The bond may be
slightly loosened, greatly weakened, or even totally broken; it may also become reinforced or strengthened. Let's
take a look at both situations.

Quantitative Blood Changes

Other than in exceptional situations (e.g., extreme hemorrhage), changes in the volume of blood are rare and usually minor. On average blood volume is 70 mL per kilogram (with one kilogram equaling 2 pounds 3.27 oz.) of body weight, or approximately 6 liters of blood for a person weighing 80 kilograms (or approximately 176.5 pounds). This ratio remains relatively constant. Yet there are people who are described as having a lot of blood and others as having not enough blood. Typically, the former are sanguine, with red faces, congested-looking, plump, with bloodshot eyes, while the latter are anemic, pale or white-complexioned, self-effacing, with lackluster eyes. The sanguine type is very connected to the material world; they enjoy the pleasures of the table and being in the company of others. They are lively, quick-tempered, and are easily angered. In contrast the more anemic type is like her own shadow; she does not always seem to be "there" and has little enthusiasm; the pleasures of life hold no appeal, and she avoids noise and the company of others. In earlier times individuals of the first type, those with excess blood, were advised to lose blood. They were the ones treated by bloodletting or the application of leeches. Anemic types, on the other hand, were advised to eat rich, fortifying foods to support the production of blood.

A man with a normal volume of blood for his body weight is usually quite conscious of his surroundings, but that consciousness will be reduced to a corresponding degree with any reduction in his blood volume. With heavy blood loss, the bond between spirit and body is weakened. The more blood lost, the more distant the injured man seems to become, ultimately losing consciousness. If the amount of blood necessary for maintaining the radiation bridge is no longer sufficient, the bond is severed. At this point the spirit separates from the body and death ensues, the death of the physical body, which can no longer be sustained and kept alive by the spirit through the radiation of the blood.

If a blood transfusion can be given soon enough, death can be avoided. In such a case, however, the benefit of the transfusion lies primarily in restoring the blood volume (quantitative modification) and only secondarily in supplying the components of the blood (qualitative modification). In fact, blood transfusions are sometimes given only as plasma (i.e., as blood removed of its usual components—red cells, white cells, etc.), simply to increase the volume of blood as efficiently as possible.

Qualitative Blood Changes

As for qualitative modifications of blood, these can be of many different kinds. Any change in oxygen content, carbon dioxide, glucose, minerals, vitamins, and so on, brings a change to the blood's composition and a corresponding change to the blood's radiation. The characteristics of the bridge are then no longer the same as previously, affecting the quality of the bond. This can result in the normal control over the body by the spirit being reduced or suspended, as partial or total loss of waking consciousness. Conversely, a positive change in any of these factors can result in a strengthening of the body-spirit bond, a subject we'll be considering later in this book. For now we'll concentrate on conditions that have an adverse effect on the body-spirit connection.

Qualitative alterations of the blood can develop if the diet does not provide all the nutrients the body needs to form blood, or if the body, on account of age or illness, is no longer able to produce the required blood radiation. Qualitative changes in the blood also occur in blood transfusions when the transfused blood does not completely match the blood group of the recipient. This can have radical effects, says *The Grail Message:*

> If a different blood group was used in the case of a blood transfusion, then the soul living in such a body would find itself prevented from fully developing its volition, would perhaps be entirely cut off from it, because with the blood of different composition the radiation also changes and is then no longer adapted to the soul. It cannot make full use of the different type of radiation or even none whatever!
>
> To the outside world such a person would then appear handicapped in his thinking and acting, because his soul cannot work properly. It can even go so far that the soul, hindered in its capacity to work, slowly severs itself from the body and leaves it altogether, which is equivalent to physical death.[1]

Blood Sugar

There are certain biological factors that can have a tremendous impact on blood, chief among them, blood sugar.

The range for blood sugar considered normal is between 70 and 110 mg of glucose per deciliter, or 100 mL of blood. Blood sugar over 120 mg is considered to be *hyperglycemia,* and under 70 mg as *hypoglycemia.* It is important to have a normal blood sugar level because sugar provides metabolic fuel—energy—for the body, and it must be present in the cells in sufficient quantities to keep the muscles, organs, and brain functioning properly. The average blood sugar level is 90 to 95 mg, and at this value the energy level is satisfactory. However, as glucose is used up, energy production declines and a feeling of physical and mental tiredness sets in. The person feels less and less able to work, and thought processes begin to slow down. At approximately 70 mg, the tiredness turns into fatigue and hunger develops. Hunger has the goal of triggering the intake of food in order to raise the blood sugar level to over 80 mg. However, if no food is consumed and the sugar level drops below 65 mg, the hunger transforms into a craving for sweet foods as the tiredness worsens, while thinking becomes cloudy.

If the hypoglycemia progresses, a variety of symptoms can develop: headache, nausea, and above all, lethargy, a feeling of rubber legs, inability to think, dizziness, and finally, loss of consciousness. Since glucose is the only source of energy for the brain, any loss of consciousness is generally explained as being a situation in which the brain has no more fuel. However, one could just as readily understand this loss of consciousness as being due to a loosening of the bond between the spirit and the body, because the center of consciousness is the spirit; the loss of consciousness is therefore a result of the inability of the spirit to use the brain after the radiation bridge has been altered due to hypoglycemia.

A change in the blood composition, and a corresponding change in blood radiation, also occurs when the blood sugar level is too high. Temporary hyperglycemia is normal after a meal rich in carbohydrates. However, the body is able to reduce the blood sugar level to normal (80–120 mg) through the secretion of insulin, the sugar-lowering hormone produced by the pancreas.

Unfortunately, insulin secretion is reduced or insufficient in certain pancreatic conditions, most notably in diabetes. Blood sugar consequently remains constantly elevated if this condition remains untreated. It can climb dangerously high after consuming carbohydrates and can lead to a hyperglycemic crisis. This abnormal blood composition can progress to the point where the person loses consciousness and falls into a diabetic coma. Thus with hyperglycemia, as we have seen with hypoglycemia, the radiation bridge is no longer available to the spirit to make it possible for it to maintain contact with the brain and the body. If the diabetic coma lasts too long, the bond becomes so weak that it finally breaks. The spirit can then no longer infuse life into the body, and death follows.

The disease of diabetes also offers another very revealing example of how blood radiation influences the bond between the spirit and the body. The diabetic's lack of insulin prevents the sugar in the blood from entering the cells. Therefore, in order to continue to function, the cells break down stored fat, which, after transformation to carbohydrates, supplies the missing fuel. However, the process of conversion of fats into carbohydrates only works effectively in the presence of glucose, which is exactly the thing that is missing in the cells of diabetics. Fat is then only incompletely broken down, and its metabolic transformation simply stops at the intermediate acid stage, characterized by the presence of ketone bodies, which are water-soluble molecules (acetone, acetoacetic acid, and beta-hydroxybutyric acid) that are produced by the liver from fatty acids during periods of low food intake (fasting) or carbohydrate restriction for cells of the body to use as energy instead of glucose.

When reserves of alkaline minerals necessary to neutralize these acids become depleted, the blood rapidly becomes more and more acidic. This is known as *keto-acidosis,* or a *ketotic crisis.* When the normal pH of the blood (7.4) becomes increasingly acidic, the character of the blood radiation also changes. Without rapid intervention the radiation becomes even more abnormal and the patient falls into a coma (keto-acedotic coma) and can die. Here too, we find another situation in which the blood radiation bond with the spirit has been greatly weakened.

Effects of Diet

Diet is another factor that can greatly influence blood composition—a subject we'll take up in greater detail later in this book. For now, let's consider the slight loosening of the bond between the spirit and the body that can occur over months and sometimes even years if the diet is continuously deficient in certain nutrients that are absolutely essential for maintaining normal blood radiation. One of the main ways this can happen is through a restrictive diet such as a lacto-vegetarian diet, in which no meat or fish is consumed, and even more so with the highly restrictive vegan diet, wherein all animal products, including eggs and milk, are omitted, and only plants in the form of cereals, legumes, fruit, and vegetables are eaten.

Over the years there have been innumerable scientific studies undertaken on the effects of diet on various aspects of health and longevity. And while there are many investigations that seem to support the advantages of lacto-vegetarian and vegan diets, for such specific health benefits as reduced HDL ("bad") cholesterol[2] and hypertension[3] and reduced risk of metabolic syndrome,[4] to name a few, there is nevertheless a vast amount of literature that points to the disadvantages of such restricted diets for most people. Vegetarian/vegan diets have been implicated in such conditions as hyperhomocysteinaemia (an abnormally high level of homocysteine in the blood), protein deficiency, anemia, decreased creatinine content in muscles, and menstrual disruption in women who undertake increased physical activity. Some of these changes may decrease the ability for performing activities that require physical effort.[5] Subnormal vitamin B_{12} status, which can lead to atherosclerosis-related diseases and cerebral atrophy, is quite prevalent in vegans and even lacto-vegetarians who eat eggs and milk products.[6]

In my practice as a naturopath, I have had many opportunities to observe the effects of vegetarian and vegan diets. Those on these kinds of restricted diets frequently give the impression of not being completely present or grounded— even though these people often interpret this condition and the feeling of distance from material goals and possessions as being signs of spiritual progress. In my opinion they have not really distanced themselves from earthly desires, only from the objects of their desires, because in reality their spirits are no longer connected as strongly with their bodies.

Hormonal Effects

In contrast with the experience of a weakened body-spirit bond, there is the opposite situation, something almost everyone has experienced at one time or another, in which the spirit is connected very strongly with the body. The spirit does not find itself drifting away from earthly reality; on the contrary it is actually more strongly connected with it and is ready to spring into action. This manifests as a feeling of anxiety or fear, wherein the spirit sees itself as being confronted by some danger. In this case as well, the radiation of the blood is significantly changed, and the effects of this change are reinforced by the secretion of various hormones, mainly adrenalin. All the physical senses are on alert, every muscle is tensed and prepared for action, and thoughts are totally focused on the present danger. In this state of extreme vigilance, the spirit is ready to intervene, whatever the danger may be and from wherever it may come. If the person reacts appropriately and escapes the difficult situation in which she finds herself, we rightly say that she displayed great "strength of spirit."

In this case the blood radiation arising in a moment of danger is therefore a help and not a hindrance. It prepares us for action and in this way supports the spirit in its protective efforts. If, on the other hand, we see this reaction as undesirable and fight to suppress it, we hinder the ability of the spirit to take action. In this situation the person becomes incapable of reacting and can therefore become completely overcome or defeated—not by the situation itself, but by the specific blood radiation that was not utilized and controlled as it could have been.

Old Age and Trauma

In the course of life, various natural processes can bring about changes in blood radiation. The weakening of the body with age may no longer permit the blood to produce radiation as strongly as it did in youth, and therefore, the body is unable to summon the same degree of heat or power as it could at a younger age. When old age, even without illness, leads to a weakening of blood radiation, the bridge becomes less and less able to retain the soul, and the body progressively loosens its bond with it. The old man finally "gives up his soul," or more precisely, his body lets go of his soul. Such is the process of a natural death, in which the soul simply and spontaneously detaches itself from the body.

Nowadays, however, fewer and fewer people die in this natural way. A rupture of the bond occurs far more commonly after the blood radiation has been weakened through serious illness or trauma of some sort (an accident, crime, war, or suicide). That a sick body can no longer produce normal blood radiation can be easily understood; body organs that are worn out or failing can no longer contribute to the formation or maintenance of a normal blood composition.

With trauma, however, changes in blood radiation can have two causes: either a sudden weakening or destruction of organs responsible for the maintenance of the blood composition, as in the case of illness, or hemorrhage due to injury. In the latter case, it is not only the loss of blood volume that weakens the bond between the body and the spirit; there is also the reduction in body heat. Significant blood loss causes a slowing of the metabolism and consequently a sharp drop in body temperature. Loss of body heat, therefore, is not only caused by prolonged exposure to cold, as occurs when someone is caught in an avalanche, falls into icy cold water, or gets lost in the mountains in winter; it can also be caused by heavy loss of blood.

Blood radiation undergoes a radical change when the body's normal temperature of 98.6 degrees Fahrenheit drops to 86 degrees. This is a very tenuous point for the body-spirit bridge—at this temperature the spirit can barely animate the body. The heart stops, breathing ceases, and the body acquires a distinctive blue color and feels cold to the touch. If the drop in temperature is due to loss of blood, a transfusion solves only one part of the problem, the quantitative aspect. But the blood also has to warm up sufficiently to permit its magnetic radiation to completely bind the spirit again, so that it can revive and reanimate the body.

In the past when this situation occurred, it was standard procedure to try to reheat the body by wrapping it in blankets, by warming the air filling the lungs, and by irrigating the stomach and abdominal cavity with warm water. However, these practices, even when all of them were combined, were not always as effective as had been hoped because the blood was reheated only secondarily, after the body had been reheated. Today we have other ways to resuscitate the person by warming the blood directly. Blood is withdrawn from an artery and its temperature is raised to 101.84 degrees Fahrenheit by flowing it through tubes immersed in warm water. Then this warmed blood is infused back into a vein. This treatment has proved much more effective, as one might expect. The reheated blood more quickly achieves the temperature required to restore power and intensity to the blood radiation, enabling the spirit to reanimate the body and the metabolism (i.e., to keep the body alive).

Sleeping and Dreaming

While in the case of death there is a complete release of the spirit, during sleep, which has been called "the little brother of death," only a certain loosening occurs. *The Grail Message* describes it this way:

> Even when the gross material body is asleep its firm union with the soul is loosened, because during sleep the body produces a different radiation which does not bind as solidly as the one required for the firm union. However, since the union still exists only a loosening takes place, but no separation. This loosening is immediately eliminated at each awakening.[7]

This loosening effect has been confirmed by the work of sleep science. When someone is sleeping, vital functions slow down—the heart beats more slowly, and blood pressure as well as body temperature drop. Signs of reduced activity in the brain are also detectable by means of an EEG. The brain, the main coordinator of all bodily functions, sends out microelectric waves that vary according to the brain's level of activity. In the waking state, the brain-wave frequency can climb as high as thirty cycles per second. The frequency begins to decline as the various phases of sleep progress, bottoming out at half a cycle per second during deep sleep.

It follows that brain activity and bodily functions are reduced during sleep. A natural consequence of the lowered metabolism is a reduction of the strength of blood radiation, which means a corresponding loosening of the bond between the spirit and the body. This loosening can actually be felt by the sleeper. While falling asleep she senses that she is gradually losing contact with her surroundings. She may feel as if she is "leaving" and may even dream of falling. This feeling of falling corresponds with the jerking movement that sometimes goes along with the loosening of the bond between the spirit and the body—something many of us have observed when watching someone who is falling asleep.

The final phase of sleep in which the bond becomes fully loosened, the phase of REM sleep (Rapid Eye Movement), can only be reached if the sleeper is lying down. In this position the spirit can withdraw from the body without danger, which is not the case if the person is sitting or standing, postures that require the presence of the spirit. In other words, without the control provided by the spirit, the body cannot remain standing or sitting on its own. To do that a certain degree of muscular tone is needed, and this is provided by the spirit.

Another fact worth noting is that REM sleep, in which the spirit-body bond is stretched the thinnest, is more quickly reached if the sleeper is in a room in which the temperature has been lowered, allowing the body temperature to fall more quickly. This helps the blood radiation to change in such a way as to facilitate the loosening of the bond. That's why most people find it easier to go to sleep with a window at least slightly open.

What Happens during
Conception and Pregnancy?

How does the blood radiation bridge form after a mother has conceived a child? When does the spirit attach itself to the fetus in the mother's womb?

As we know the earthly cloak is only the material vessel of the spirit; the origin of the spirit is not to be found within it. It exists eternally, beyond the appearance of the physical body, which shelters it. The body only gradually takes on its definitive form, a form adapted to the individual spirit in the course of its development during pregnancy, childhood, and right up to adolescence.

But during the earliest stages of development, the embryo cannot itself provide a bridge for the spirit since the volume of blood is still quite small and has not yet acquired its normal composition. Considering that the blood radiation of an adult body at the end of life is no longer capable of binding to the spirit, how could an embryo that measures only a few centimeters do so, especially when its organs are still developing and cannot actively participate in the formation of blood?

Nevertheless, the bond between the spirit and the fetus needs to take place fairly early on because the fetus is being prepared for that specific spirit. The formation of the body must not only follow its genetic code, it must also conform to the characteristics of the spirit that will inhabit it. So, since the fetus does not yet produce sufficient blood radiation, what bridge can the awaiting spirit use to connect with its tiny developing body? The answer to this question follows from our understanding of blood radiation. As the bridge can only be formed by blood radiation, it becomes obvious that it must be the blood that is closest at hand, which is always there: the blood of the mother.

It must be stressed here that contrary to widely held belief, it is not the blood of the mother herself that flows through the fetus. At no time, other than perhaps through some accident, does the blood of the mother cross over into the circulatory system of the developing fetus. Each has her own separate circulatory system. To be sure the mother's blood infuses and "feeds" the placenta and through it nourishes the fetus, but the two systems of blood flow always remain separate.

It is the radiation of the mother's blood, therefore, that permits the spirit of the unborn child to bind with the body being prepared for it by the mother. This is still only a bonding and not yet the actual incarnation, because the embryo, in its early stages of development, does not yet have the human form capable of receiving a spirit.

An incarnation can only take place when the fetus and its blood have developed sufficiently to be able to provide the spirit with a dwelling as well as the required bridge. In reality, during the first days following conception, the embryo is only a mass of multiplying cells that passes through all the stages of evolution that animal species have undergone in the course of millennia. Thus initially it resembles a sea creature, a mollusk or a fish, and at this stage it even has primitive gill structures. Next it takes on the form of an amphibian; then a land animal, climbing further up the chain of development to the mammal, right up to the primate, and finally achieving human form. It is only at the end of the first month of pregnancy that the organs of the fetus start to develop their structure and take on human form. This development acquires more detail during the two or three months that follow, up to approximately the middle of the pregnancy. At this time, from the fourth month on, the organs of the fetus are almost identical to those of a newborn, right down to their basic structure.

The blood vessels develop relatively early, and the heart starts pulsing on the twenty-fourth day of gestation, but only truly beats from about the twenty-ninth day on. Blood is present in the blood vessels but does not circulate in these early days. As well, the blood does not yet have its final composition. The red blood cells begin to form at the third week, and interestingly have a nucleus that later disappears and is not present in the final red blood cells. In the fourth week, red blood cells are produced by the mesenchymal tissue and by the endothelium of the blood vessels of the fetus. They are also produced in the liver from the sixth week and by the spleen and lymphatic tissue from the third month on.

All the organs that participate in the formation of blood are active from the fourth month on. By this time the blood of the fetus has acquired a sufficiently developed composition to produce a radiation capable of binding the spirit. Consequently it is at this time, in the middle of the pregnancy, when the incarnation of the spirit in the developing human body is able to take place. As *The Grail Message* states:

> The incarnation, that is, the entrance of the soul, takes place about the middle of pregnancy. The growing state of maturity, both of the expectant mother and of the soul preparing to incarnate, also produces a special and more earthly tie. This comprises radiations created by their

mutual state of maturity, which irresistibly strive towards one another in natural release. These radiations increase more and more and unite the soul and the expectant mother ever more closely in their longing for each other, until finally, when the developing body in the mother's womb has reached a certain maturity, the soul is literally absorbed by it.

The moment when the soul enters, or is being absorbed, naturally brings about the first shock to the little body, which shows itself in twitchings called the first movements of the child. When this occurs the expectant mother very often experiences a change in her inner feelings, either uplifting or oppressive according to the kind of soul that has entered.[8]

Thus the spirit does not incarnate at the time of fertilization and conception, nor does it incarnate at the moment of birth; it does during the middle of the pregnancy, at about four or four-and-a-half months. With its entry into the body, the spirit can put its personal stamp much more strongly on its physical development, because the bond that previously had been quite loose is now strengthened and is about to become tight. This will have repercussions not only for the further development of the organs, which continue to develop during the second half of pregnancy, but also for the formation of the blood, which now can become even more specific to the nature of the incarnated spirit.

By midterm the radiation of the mother's blood has completed its role as the temporary bridge for the spirit of the unborn child. Without this temporary bridge, the connection with the developing body would have been impossible. The bridge is therefore indispensable, and we can predict with certainty the impossibility of bringing to term, even with the aid of sophisticated technology, a test-tube baby in the literal sense of this term (i.e., outside of the womb of the mother). The presence of a radiation bridge is an absolute necessity.

Psychic Parasites

Let's turn our attention to a special situation in which a spirit in the beyond misappropriates blood radiation not destined for it, like a parasite. We have just seen that a similar situation exists when the spirit of the child waiting to incarnate first uses the radiation of the blood of its mother to connect with its future body. This is necessary and normal for human beings. However, it can happen, as we shall soon see, that a spirit from the beyond can also use this means of approach without actually undergoing an earthly incarnation.

A spirit in the beyond cannot connect with just anyone's blood. There has to be an affinity with the blood radiation of the person involved. It was mentioned in the previous section that the radiation of the blood has to resemble the radiation of the spirit wishing to enter the world of matter. In the case of pregnancy, the spirit of the child awaiting to incarnate can, in principle, only be one with an affinity to the spirit of the mother; a spiritual affinity, often falsely attributed to physical heredity, must exist. In reality DNA and genetics play a role only for the physical body because the spirit preexists the body. Heredity is only physical; there is no such thing as spiritual heredity. Any similarity other than physical between parents and children is due to the fact that parents attract spirits with characteristics similar to their own that then become their offspring. As well the affinity between the mother and the child does not imply that the blood type of the child has to be the same as that of the mother, because the known blood types are only one of the many characteristics of blood.

In cases of psychic blood parasites, we have a situation in which a spirit from the beyond attaches to the blood radiation of a person as a means of manifesting on the earthly plane in order to cause ghostly phenomena such as the moving of objects, knocking, and so on. When these manifestations occur, the entire household can become completely terrorized by phenomena such as doors opening by themselves, objects mysteriously changing place or dropping on the floor and breaking, curtains moving without any air movement, and knocking sounds or other strange noises. All these phenomena have one thing in common: they take place in the presence of one particular person. Constant observation of the person involved never reveals any voluntary involvement on their part in the moving or knocking, and so the cause of the strange manifestations is a mystery, especially since such phenomena often stop after a few weeks or months for no apparent reason.

The explanation for this phenomenon can be found in *The Grail Message:* it has to do with the particular nature of the blood radiation of the person—a girl, in the following excerpt—whose presence provides a host environment for the spirit from the beyond:

> In the house concerned a *human spirit* may be *earthbound* through some cause or other; for *in all cases* it can only be

a question of *human spirits* which have departed from the earth. Demons or the like are utterly out of the question in this matter.

Through some deed such a human spirit is perhaps bound to the house or only to the place, the spot. Thus it need not necessarily have done something during *the period* when the house existed, but it may have already been *before* then, at or near the spot where the house now stands.

Sometimes this spirit is tied to the place for decades or centuries, either through a murder or through some grave act of negligence, through harming some other person as well as through other happenings, many of which can bind a person.

Therefore it is not absolutely necessary for it to be connected with the people inhabiting the house *now.* Despite its perpetual presence in the house it has at all events never before had an opportunity enabling it to manifest itself in the gross material on earth, which *now only* takes place through the girl on account of her special, *but also only present,* peculiarity.

This peculiarity of the girl is a matter all by itself, which merely gives the spirit the opportunity of expressing its volition in the gross material world in a certain way. It has otherwise nothing to do with the spirit.

The cause of the peculiarity lies in the radiation of her blood at that time, the instant it has *a very definite composition.* It is *from this* that the human spirit without a gross material earth cloak derives strength for carrying out its desires to make itself conspicuous, which often develop into irksome bad behaviour.

As I have once already pointed out every person has different blood radiations, and this blood composition is changed several times during life on earth, whereby the type of radiation of the blood also changes at the same time. Thus in most cases the singular effect some persons exercise in being able to set free the unusual happenings occurs over a very definite period only, i.e., *temporarily*. There is hardly a single case where it lasts during the whole earth life. Sometimes it continues only for weeks or months, but seldom for years.

Therefore when such a happening suddenly ceases this does not prove that the spirit concerned no longer exists or is released, but in most cases it has suddenly no further possibility of making itself conspicuous in such a crude way.[9]

This sudden cessation of the paranormal phenomena comes about due to another alteration in the blood composition of the host, and the resulting changed blood radiation no longer provides a bridge for the disincarnate spirit.

The Phenomenon of Possession

The case just described could be considered annoying but relatively harmless. There are much more serious situations that can develop in which a disincarnate spirit is not satisfied with simply drawing from the power of the blood radiation of a host to enable itself to act in the material world; rather, it seeks to use the blood radiation of a host to literally work through this body in the gross material plane (i.e., to possess it).

In such a case, a spirit in the beyond uses the host's blood radiation bridge to take possession of his body and to make use of it for its own ends. The body is indeed used by the spirit, but in this case by a spirit who is not the rightful owner of that physical body. The usurper cannot, of course, drive out the rightful owner of the body completely, otherwise the body would cease to be animated and would die, because the disincarnate spirit is not connected closely enough to the body to keep it alive on its own.

Taking possession of a body is not an easy thing to do because there not only needs to be a blood radiation that suits the disincarnate spirit, there also has to be a certain weakness and lack of resistance on the part of the host. However, no one is left without some form of protection from these kinds of attempts by spirits from the beyond. Simple defensive actions, most often subconscious, suffice to protect against possession. Protection is therefore provided by keeping a consistent spiritual vigilance and by the strong blood radiation that results from this watchfulness.

The possession of a body can be more or less complete. It is logical that possession takes place primarily at the level of the brain, because it controls the entire body. The brain, being a tool of the spirit, will be used at one moment by the disincarnate spirit, and in the next by its rightful spirit/host when the one releases control to the other, or simultaneously when the two spirits fight for control of the brain. This inevitably results in a great confusion of thoughts, words, and actions, and this confusion can be attributed to the fact that there are two different users working with the same tool. To return to our metaphor of the brain as a computer, it is as though two different persons are using the same computer at the same time, but with different programs.

This overriding of the host's brain causes derangement, which contributes to even greater confusion. This manifests in different ways, varying greatly according to the nature of the individual case and circumstances. It could manifest as a difficulty paying attention and concentrating; a lack of logic; disturbed, broken, or incoherent speech; or absentmindedness, withdrawal, and passivity. It could also manifest as agitation, frenzied behavior, aggressiveness, inconsistency, reacting unpredictably, bizarre or contradictory behavior, and obsessive thoughts.

According to the type and degree of possession, the abnormal behavior could be temporary or may become permanent. From the outside the behavior of the person appears totally bizarre. It is for this reason that he is treated as insane; however, the root of this "insanity" lies in the difficulty of the rightful spirit to act in a normal way because of the battle being waged between the two spirits, and in the manifestations of the possessing spirit, which are inconsistent with the thinking and personality of the owner of the body.

Possession is not always a matter of just one spirit from the beyond; several spirits can fight over the control of a brain. To the observer the person affected can appear to change personality several times over the course of a single day. Thus he may be gentle and considerate in one moment, then impulsive or violent in another; or refined and cultivated, then coarse and crude. He can appear to have a profound knowledge about a certain subject and then be totally ignorant of it later. In certain cases one can count up to a dozen different personalities in a single patient. For a medical doctor or psychiatrist, these are only different roles being played by a single person—the rightful owner of the brain. In reality what's happening is a real battle among any number of disincarnate spirits over the use of the brain of the host, who is the rightful owner of the brain.

The medical term for this is schizophrenia, which actually corresponds perfectly with the explanation given for possession, with the exception of one central factor: the cause of this condition.

Here is a medical definition of schizophrenia, to which I have added some commentary in brackets:

> Schizophrenia is an endogenous complaint of unknown origin, mainly characterized by a splitting of the personality, with mental-verbal disassociation and wild, confused thoughts [two spirits battling over one brain], giving the impression of being under the influence of alien forces [the disincarnated spirit or spirits]; a feeling of detachment from the self [the rightful spirit being pushed out]; the experience of feelings not belonging to the patient [those of the other spirit]; loss of contact with reality [the reality of the rightful spirit versus the reality lived by the intruder]; in general, without reduction of lucidity or irreversible deterioration of the intellect [not a disease of the brain but rather a conflict over control of the brain].[10]

Given that today most people are ignorant of the concept of blood radiation, and that the distinction between spirit and body is generally not well known (or is even rejected), numerous people have been described as incurably insane when in reality they are possessed and could benefit greatly from treatment, that treatment consisting of changing the composition of the blood in such a way that the resulting new blood radiation would enable the person's own spirit to express itself fully, unhindered by any interference from another spirit.*

In the following chapters we will take a closer look at blood's influence on the spirit. A better understanding of this relationship will take us one step closer to learning how to modify our blood radiation so that our spirit can be optimized.

---

*Clearly, this type of treatment is only possible when the brain is healthy. It is another matter when the symptoms of mental illness are due to a disease of the brain itself.

FIVE

∽

Blood's Influence on the Spirit

Absolute harmony must also prevail in the composition of the radiations of the human body in order to provide the spirit with the best means for its protection, development and advancement, such as are meant for it in the normal course of development in Creation.

ABD-RU-SHIN, *IN THE LIGHT OF TRUTH: THE GRAIL MESSAGE*

The main task of the blood consists of offering the spirit the radiation that it requires. This radiant energy depends on the composition of the blood; therefore, each blood component— red blood cells, proteins, minerals, and so on—plays a role in the formation of the overall radiation of the blood. Healthy blood, which contains all these components in certain quantities, offers the spirit what it needs. If the levels of the different components change, the blood radiation also changes. If one of the substances needed for forming healthy blood is missing, then the radiation is affected and the spirit is deprived of its optimal radiation. If, on the other hand, some substance suddenly appears in the blood that normally is not a part of blood composition—for instance, poison in some form—then the blood radiation is again changed, but in a way that the spirit does not recognize. Depending on the substance, the resulting change to the blood could merely throw the person a little off balance, or she could become completely disturbed and unsettled. If the poisoning is severe enough, the connection between the spirit and the body could be at risk.

The nature, properties, and "color" of the blood affect its radiation and contribute to providing the spirit with what it needs for its activity in the material world and for the absorption of impressions and information from its earthly surroundings. Whatever qualitative changes the blood undergoes affect the blood's radiation and thereby affect this perceptive ability of the spirit, such that the way the spirit sees things, and even the spirit's awareness of itself, undergoes a change.

The gateway or bridge that the blood radiation provides is absolutely necessary for the spirit. It is the only pathway by which it can gather impressions and information from the body.

The perceptions of the spirit depend on the blood radiation much like the way someone who wears glasses depends on those glasses to see clearly. Anyone who wears glasses sees the world as a result of the particular characteristics of the corrective prescription of those glasses—much like our unique blood radiation informs our view of the world. If the lenses are made for close up, as reading glasses are, then the vision will not be the same as with a pair of distance glasses, whose lenses have a different prescription in order to enable the wearer to see great distances. In addition, if the lenses are strongly tinted, the world will be perceived as being the color of that tint, although in reality it is not that color. The same is true of the blood radiation.

Spirit's Perceptual Lens

The influence of blood radiation on the spirit of a person cannot be underestimated. For example, when the blood sugar level is normal, the person "feels comfortable in his skin." He has drive and is dynamic and enterprising. But when the glucose content falls, the person feels tired and unwell. Not only is there no energy, but his entire view of the world also changes. Where just a short while ago everything was rosy, now the world seems gray or even truly dark. A person in a hypoglycemic crisis becomes anxious, fearful of all kinds of things not seen as frightening by those around him, and simple questions become insurmountable problems. Fears and problems that weren't there before the hypoglycemic crisis suddenly become realities that seem unsolvable. No amount of reasoning or encouragement is of any help. This new view of "reality" settles in so strongly that the person might forget that only a short time ago, he felt perfectly well and happy, without a care in the world. Then he eats and the blood sugar level returns to normal, anxiety lifts, the world again becomes beautiful and simple as before. Problems and fears disappear, and the person will wonder why everything looked so dark just a few moments ago and will laugh at himself.

Drugs and Alcohol

It is well known that one's state of consciousness is affected by the abuse of mind-altering substances such as alcohol. When someone gets drunk, we say she is not her "normal self"—her perception and behavior change according to her altered awareness of reality. When the person's blood alcohol level drops back to normal and she sobers up, her blood radiation also returns to normal. Her spirit then perceives her surroundings in the accustomed way and acts "normal."

What the person said and did under the influence of alcohol is often regretted afterward. It is said she was "under the influence." Indeed, she was not herself, given that her blood radiation had been altered by the presence of alcohol. If she had "kept a clear head" (i.e., if her spirit had not lost control over her brain and body), her words and actions would have been quite different. However, with her particular blood radiation having been affected by the alcohol, her spirit could not fully assert itself. It is as if it had been pushed aside, and the self-control, the sense of morality and dignity—attributes of the spirit, not the brain—were rendered inactive for the duration of time she was drunk.

Every drug, whether it be alcohol, tobacco, marijuana, heroin, cocaine, prescription drugs, or whatever other mind-altering substance yet to be discovered or created, whether taken medically or not, separately or as a cocktail, alters the blood radiation in a particular way and leads to varying repercussions on the perceptions of the spirit.

Drug-induced changes are widely known, and anyone taking drugs is looking for a certain high (or a suppressed state), with the main goal being to detach from or alter reality. If the person is not happy with her perception of the world as mediated by her normal blood radiation, then she can change it by taking a drug selected for the effects that she wants to have. The drug overrides her spirit's volition, with the consequences being the person is operating in an altered state of reality.

Heavy Metal Overload

Besides drugs, which are taken intentionally, there are any number of substances that can get into the blood without our ever knowing it and cause our blood radiation to become altered, thereby affecting the perceptions of the spirit. Among the most insidious blood-altering substances to be found in our modern-day environment are heavy metals such as lead, mercury, arsenic, aluminum, and so on, which can originate in the air, the water, or the soil.

Let's consider lead, for example. Lead poisoning leads to various physical symptoms such as colic, encephalopathy (brain dysfunction), anemia, and neuropathy[1] but also different psychic symptoms such as nightmares, hallucinations, and delusions; a person may see, hear, or smell things that are not there.

Notably, the level of lead, as well as other heavy metals, is generally much higher in the blood of criminals. According to a study undertaken in Switzerland, the lead concentration in the blood of prisoners is twice as high as in other population groups.[2] Lead toxicity cannot, of course, be held solely responsible for the malicious behavior of incarcerated persons;

lead does not create criminals, but in changing the blood radiation, it contributes to a clouded perception and judgment.

Copper, a substance that is beneficial in small quantities, can have detrimental effects on blood radiation at higher doses. The normal blood level of copper is between 64 and 143 micrograms per 100 grams of blood. If the level of copper increases beyond this normal range (for example, as a result of eating acid foods cooked in uncoated copper cookware or from exposure to excess copper in drinking water or other environmental sources), symptoms can include vomiting, hematemesis (vomiting of blood), hypotension (low blood pressure), melena (black, tarry feces), coma, jaundice, and gastrointestinal distress.[3] With this kind of poison in the blood, everything the spirit sees makes it irritable and hot-tempered, depressed and paranoid.

To counteract this condition and lower the copper content of the blood, we use its antagonist, zinc. Taking zinc gets rid of the surplus copper and, at the same time, changes the blood radiation and the general condition of the patient. His usual temperament returns; he once again can feel joyful and loving toward those around him.

Whatever the state of the blood radiation, the human spirit always retains its faculty of freedom of choice; it can try to remain calm and amicable at any given moment. This ability is seriously challenged, however, when there is an excess of any heavy metal, or any other substance that disturbs the blood radiation.

It is important to realize that sensitivity to various substances, dietary or otherwise, varies from one person to the next. A substance that can be perfectly well tolerated by a great number of people can cause serious difficulties for others, until the real cause of their condition is discovered.

ADD/ADHD

Since the beginning of the twentieth century, a new and unusual pattern of behavior has been observed among children, which has led many of these young people to delinquency. The condition, ADHD, or attention deficit hyperactivity disorder (or ADD, attention deficit disorder), causes the child to be hyperactive, unable to sit still, in constant motion. These children seem to have to put their hands on everything, and they talk too much. Their power of concentration is low and they are easily distracted. They cannot keep to one activity and frequently jump from one thing to another and end up finishing nothing. They are careless, absent-minded, and neglectful. Despite a great need for affection, they have great difficulty establishing relationships, mostly because of their unpredictable, stubborn, and unmanageable nature. Lying and contemptuous, they are finally rejected by those around them.

The hyperactivity that characterizes these children, along with their resistance to any change in surroundings, makes them suspicious, hostile, and aggressive. They tease and bully other children. There is constant fighting and hitting. The violence can also be directed against objects: toys are destroyed, furniture and glass broken. During violent episodes of this kind, the child has absolutely no control over his actions, seeming to have hardly any awareness of what he's doing, and does not remember anything afterward. If you catch these children red-handed and try to reason with them, they seem distant. No comment or threat gets through to them. They are not really reachable and, because of that, they seem incorrigible. It is sometimes said these children act as if they are being driven by someone else. The core of their personality, their spirit, does not seem to be present and in control. Their body acts on its own, as if controlled by something stronger than their spirit.

Parents, teachers, and therapists who sought to help these children gradually became aware that they were dealing with something quite specific, and that the standard explanations for maladjustment, such as rebellion, spoiling, and so on, did not apply to these children. Later on it was discovered that the behavioral disturbances started to show up when the diet was changed. The conclusion was that some type of food played a part in the problem. But which food or substances was it? Nobody knew. Finally, Hertha Hafer, a German pharmacist, discovered the culprit: phosphate, a preservative found in meat and sausages, also used as a flavor enhancer in soups and colas, and as an anticaking agent.[4] When the diet no longer contains phosphates, a child displaying this syndrome normalizes, becoming more present and self-aware.

With a condition such as ADHD/ADD, a diet without phosphates is adopted. It takes about three days before all symptoms disappear and for the blood radiation to normalize. Taking specific remedies can bring about an even quicker effect. In addition to certain pharmaceuticals, ordinary wine vinegar can neutralize phosphates, sometimes within half an hour, even in the middle of an attack.

A young person with ADHD/ADD who regularly consumes

fast food and colas might also display antisocial behavior or seek refuge in drugs. But if he follows a strict diet, without phosphates, he can likely correct the abnormal blood radiation and bring about a more balanced mental, physical, and spiritual state.

Vitamin and Mineral Deficiencies

As suggested in chapter 4 (see "Effects of Diet"), significant changes in blood radiation, and consequently one's spiritual potential, can result from an absence of substances necessary for normal blood composition, such as certain vitamins and minerals.

A study was conducted in which subjects were fed a normal diet but with total restriction of vitamin B_1 (i.e., thiamin). At the end of three months, all the subjects had become irritable, depressed, and worried that some misfortune might befall them. Some even began to feel suicidal. Six months into the experiment, the physical effects became painful (headache, nausea, severe vomiting). At this point vitamin B_1 was added to the subjects' diet, but without informing the trial subjects, in order to avoid any placebo effect. After only a few days, the trial subjects rediscovered their joy of life and clarity of spirit and became friendly, cooperative, and enthusiastic.[5]

That all the subjects in this experiment became worried that something might happen to them (although there was really nothing wrong), and that this fear disappeared shortly after the subjects were given vitamin B_1, clearly shows that it was the perception of the spirit and not something within the spirit itself, that was the root of the problem. Certainly, for the trial subjects themselves, the fear was perfectly real, and they had to struggle to overcome it. This cannot be compared to real fear in the face of real danger. In the course of the experiment, the spirits of the volunteers were not changed by the lack of vitamin B_1; the subjects lost neither their personal attributes nor their abilities. Something material like a vitamin does not have the power to directly affect something nonmaterial like a spirit. It was the change in blood radiation—the body's bridge to the spirit—that was altered as a result of the missing nutrient, vitamin B_1.

Magnesium provides another good example of how this can happen. A slight magnesium deficiency makes one irritable, nervous, sensitive to noise, excitable, and anxious. A greater deficiency can be even more serious, so much so that the subject becomes disoriented, wildly excited, and aggressive. With alcoholics the terrifying hallucinations of the DTs, delirium tremens, along with the changes in the brain, appear to result in large part from the lack of magnesium caused by alcohol consumption. The angry and violent behavior disappears quickly if we supply the missing magnesium to reestablish normal blood radiation.

Lithium, another mineral, is used in psychiatry to bring the behavior of manic depressives into balance. The lithium requirement of the body is extremely low. With a person in good health, ingested lithium is quickly eliminated in the urine, whereas manic depressives retain it, even high quantities, and only start to eliminate it when they begin to feel better. It is as if the body wants to conserve the lithium it requires in order to keep enough in reserve in the blood. Since food contains very little lithium, it must be given as a supplement to these persons, and in significant quantities (50 to 1,500 mg daily). The body uses it to maintain the blood radiation, which the spirit needs in order to keep control over the body. In fact, when the blood level of lithium reaches a sufficient level, recovery comes at the end of one to two weeks. In general, these patients take lithium all the time as a preventive measure, although this really would only be necessary if the lithium content of the blood again declined.

The Role of the Endocrine Glands

The endocrine system plays a fundamental role in blood radiation. The pineal gland, pituitary gland, ovaries, testes, thyroid gland, parathyroid gland, hypothalamus, and adrenal glands comprise the major glands of the endocrine system. These glands are called *endocrine* because their secretions—hormones—are emptied directly into the blood. This contrasts with the exocrine glands—the sweat glands, salivary glands, mammary glands, and liver—which secrete their essential products by way of a duct to some environment external to itself, either inside the body or on a surface of the body (e.g., digestive juices into the intestine, perspiration of the sweat glands onto the skin). The importance of hormones is still insufficiently understood, yet they are determining factors for blood radiation and the potentials of the spirit.

We assume that the brain is the great control center where everything starts and on which everything depends. However, without the thyroid gland or its secretions, a person cannot think at all; she has no feelings, no needs or desires, nor any intellectual life. The brain and sensory nerves would be asleep without the thyroid and its secretions. The eyes see, the ears hear, but the person is as if deaf and dumb. In medicine such a person is referred to as being in a vegetative state. The absence of thyroid hormones in the blood prevents the spirit from using the brain. The tool is there, but the user appears to be absent, disconnected, unplugged. This deficiency in the blood radiation of the person prevents her from using this tool. Simply supplying the missing thyroid hormone will remedy this situation. The patient awakens from her stupor; she can feel, take notice, react, and think.

The activity of the endocrine glands changes over time. The thymus, for instance, which lies at the base of the neck, is mostly active during childhood, but with adolescence it begins to atrophy and disappear. The sex glands do not assume their full activity until puberty and are less active toward the end of life. These changes, as well all those that the body undergoes during childhood, adolescence, adulthood, and old age, see to it that the blood composition changes over time, providing different blood radiations for the different stages of life.

To this must be added the fact that at birth each person receives a body whose organs may be either stronger or weaker because of heredity. These differences from one person to the next naturally bring about diverse possibilities for the development of the blood. Whatever blood radiation that results from one's heredity provides a unique means by which each person can express himself. These differences have long been observed and form the basis for classifying humans into groupings of similar characteristics: the four temperaments.

The Four Temperaments

The ancient concept of the four temperaments was a medical theory proposed by Hippocrates, who suggested that there are four fundamental personality types: sanguine (pleasure-seeking and sociable), choleric (ambitious and leaderlike), melancholic (analytical and quiet), and phlegmatic (relaxed and peaceful). Most formulations include the possibility of mixtures of the types. The association of these temperaments with blood has long been recognized and is found in such expressions as a person being "hot-blooded," "cold-blooded," and so on.

We each inherit a temperament or a combination of temperaments. However, during the course of life, every human being, because of changes in blood radiation, goes through four major stages in life that are colored by the characteristics of one or other of the four temperaments. The temperaments are then grouped into four age periods that, along with the different kinds of blood radiation that go along with them, offer the spirit different potentials for its sojourn on Earth.

The sanguine temperament corresponds to childhood. It is seen in the joy of life, enthusiasm, light-heartedness, spontaneity, and effervescence. It is life without cares, living from one day to the next. One could say that the spirit takes things lightly and without any sense of responsibility. And that is the way it really is, because childhood is the time when the spirit does nothing other than discover the world into which it finds itself incarnated. Before it has understood how everything works by living through life's experiences, it can obviously not yet act with a true sense of responsibility. Only upon entering adolescence will its apprenticeship have been sufficient to enable it to begin to act more consciously, in preparation for adulthood.

Then the temperament changes and the spirit is bathed in the blood radiation of the melancholic temperament. The melancholic period of adolescence, with its nostalgic daydreams, leads young men and women to an awareness of the serious side of life and to bit by bit prepare for earthly activity. With the awakening of the sex glands in adolescence, the blood radiation changes substantially. By means of the new radiation bridge now offered to it, the spirit establishes a far closer contact with reality. It ceases to flit about in life the way it had done during childhood and sees ever more clearly the responsibility that it must assume for its actions. The ardent yearning and striving after high ideals typical of this phase of life helps the future adults to direct their actions in a harmonious and beneficial way.

Strictly speaking, true earthly activity does not begin until the end of adolescence and the beginning of the choleric temperament of the adult. With the period of learning and the awakening of consciousness complete, the spirit can now start to give concrete expression to its will in earthly life. It puts its own stamp on its environment, transforms it, and begins to achieve things of its own and see the results. The "excitable" blood of the choleric temperament pushes toward action and is eager to get going and get things done. The spirit has no time or inclination for a passive life; it seeks to build as long as it is on the Earth.

Toward the end of life, the spirit has to learn to leave behind everything earthly, which it will soon be doing, and turn toward higher pursuits. The phlegmatic temperament that sets in with aging contributes to this progressive loosening. The need to affirm itself and be active in the material world decreases and is replaced by a profound desire to understand the meaning of life itself. Activity gives way to quiet meditation on the experiences gained from life and past achievements. When the period of phlegmatic temperament is fully experienced, death can be faced without fear, and the spirit can easily detach itself from its earthly cloak.

Through the different temperaments, the spirit makes use of the different blood radiations to enable it to take the best advantage of life.

Blood Radiation and Depression

Knowledge of the relationship between temperament and blood radiation can provide us with an approach for the treatment of depression and manic depression.

In the past the term *melancholy* was used to describe what we today call depression. Could there be a relationship between depression and the melancholic temperament or, more accurately, the kind of blood radiation that dominates with the melancholic temperament?

Although depression is not a particular characteristic of the melancholic temperament, it can nevertheless be said that people with a melancholic temperament are more easily subject to depression. Could it not also be said that a person with depression displays symptoms that resemble, in an exaggerated way, the peculiarities of the melancholic temperament, only distorted and intensified? With depression the serious look of someone with a melancholic temperament is not just thoughtful reflection, it becomes a feeling of oppression; day-dreaming changes into morbid analyzing, nostalgia changes into anxiety, and sadness into discouragement and fear. In manic-depressives episodes of depression alternate with mania, which appears as a caricature of the sanguine temperament. The vivacity of this temperament, full of joie de vivre, is transformed into hyperactivity and excitability; living one day at a time turns into carelessness; spontaneity becomes inconsistency and irresponsibility.

The treatment of these two illnesses, depression and manic depression, must then be focused on changing the blood radiation, with the aim of reestablishing a blood composition in keeping with the true nature of the person's temperament and not an exaggerated version of it. Note that we use the term *de-pression,* which implies a reduction of pressure. What sort of pressure is meant by this? Observation of depressed people leads us to use this term because their entire manner, the way they look, what radiates from them, demonstrates a lack of pressure. It is obviously not blood pressure nor any supposed pressure in the nervous system, but rather an inner pressure resulting from the *ex-pression* of the will (i.e., the outward pressure we exert on our surroundings through the way we go about our lives). Our words and our actions make an *im-pression* on those around us.

We have already noted that it is the spirit that plays a central role in expressing the will and the personality. We can certainly express something purely intellectually, making corresponding facial expressions and gestures, but the effect is completely different when we express something with the warmth and vitality generated with the full participation of the spirit.

It is the same as the difference between a mere "thanks" out of politeness and a sincere "thank-you" coming from the bottom of the heart.

In a depressed person, the blood radiation does not provide a sufficient bridge for the spirit to act with its full power to exert its impressions on the person as well as to counterbalance or equalize pressure coming from the outside. On the contrary the spirit of the depressed person is not just exposed to external pressure, it is overwhelmed by it, thereby giving rise to anxiety, despair, and a sense of resignation. It no longer feels on top of things and, for the moment, rightly so. A certain something is missing from the blood radiation.

Psychotherapy cannot succeed until the spirit can be reached and, in responding, it alters the blood radiation, as we shall see in the next chapter. However, treatment at the level of the blood is also possible. This consists of a correction or readaptation of the blood radiation to the needs of the spirit, so that it can again assert itself and express all its abilities.

Clairvoyance

So far we have seen that blood radiation consists of different kinds of radiation, just as the blood consists of different components. In other words each specific blood radiation has a corresponding color, and the sum total of these colors results in the complete spectrum of blood radiation. Healthy blood contains all the colors, and thus everything it needs is placed at the disposal of the spirit. But the proportions of the different colors differ in the blood of one person to the next, and so the many possible color combinations form an endless variety of different bridges, corresponding to the diversity of human spirits. Some blood radiations may contain, for instance, much green and yellow but very little blue, while in another person blue and purple might predominate.

Beyond the different proportions of color entering into the different compositions of radiations, blood can also differ through the quality of the colors. These can be pure and have a more or less radiant glow. They can be dark or, alternatively, very bright and lively. As one could easily imagine, a dull yellow radiation does not offer the same possibilities as that of a sparkling golden yellow. To explain the difference that exists between the type and quality of radiations as expressed by different colors, let us turn to the phenomenon of clairvoyance.

A clairvoyant is a person who can see what is happening in planes of Creation that lie beyond the dense matter that is visible to our earthly eyes. In general one assumes that clairvoyance is a special ability of the spirit of the clairvoyant person. In reality, clairvoyance is not an ability of the spirit, but rather it depends on a special type of blood radiation. This can change in the course of time with alterations of the blood and its radiation. This explains why clairvoyance can appear suddenly, can decrease, or can even disappear entirely. Most people, because of their blood radiation, can only see with the eyes of their earthly body. But in addition to its physical body, the incarnated spirit carries cloaks, or bodies, of the various planes that the spirit has traveled through on its way to Earth. These bodies all possess sensory organs, exactly like the earthly body, including eyes. If they are not active, it is because normally only the sensory organs corresponding to the plane in which the spirit finds itself now are active and working. Some people, however, have a special kind of blood radiation that permits them to see with the eyes of their ethereal body. This special kind of radiation provides a connection with the spirit, opening the eyes of the ethereal body, thereby paving the way for the spirit of the clairvoyant to gain access to something more.

The seeing of clairvoyants differs greatly from one to another. They do not all see the same thing, because they are seeing with "eyes" of different kinds. For some their seeing reaches into the astral plane; for others to fine matter or at least to a certain level of that plane. The unique faculty of clairvoyance depends on a very specific kind of blood radiation, but that which can actually be seen depends on the *quality* of these radiations. The finer and purer the blood radiations, the higher the plane or sphere that can be seen—meaning that the "eyes" being used for the seeing are those of the higher ethereal body of the clairvoyant.

Rightly understood this fineness and purity of blood radiation can naturally not be obtained merely through a certain type of diet or through the supply of certain substances into the blood. The deciding factor is the spirit. It plays, as we shall see in the next chapter, a determining role in the development of the blood radiation.

~

SIX

The Spirit's Influence on the Blood

Man on earth should cherish his body as property entrusted to him, and strive to achieve healthy harmony between spirit and body.

ABD-RU-SHIN, *IN THE LIGHT OF TRUTH: THE GRAIL MESSAGE*

As we have seen, blood radiation appears to be determined by such physical factors as heredity, diet, and the physical condition of the organs of the body. However, this is only part of the picture. The spirit influences blood radiation in many ways, always changing and adapting it to its present state, giving it attributes corresponding with its own. This constant adaptation of the blood radiation to the current state and will of the spirit is essential because the spirit can only fully experience its earthly incarnation through the physical body. The feelings and wishes of the spirit have to be expressed through the body so that it can gain the desired experiences in the earthly plane. Change to the blood radiation by the spirit is the means to this end, causing corresponding changes at the level of the physical body.

The Evolution of the Human Spirit

Research into the origins of human beings has shown that humans descended from apelike animals. Even though the evolution of humans from creatures similar to large apes is a widely accepted theory, scientists still ask themselves how the qualitative leap from the rudimentary psyche of the great apes to the highly developed one of human beings came about. When we accept that the spirit is not of the same nature as the body, that it is the spirit that is the true nature of human beings, this question is answered. What descended from the apelike animal is the physical body of man, his outermost cloak, his tool, but not his spirit, which is his central driving force. Until the appearance of the first human on Earth, there were only animal souls incarnated in the bodies of the great apes. After the incarnation of the first human spirits, however, this bodily form further developed and ennobled itself under the influence of the spirit. It lost its animal appearance, and a body with human characteristics developed.

Humans, then, descended from apelike animals, but even so, despite certain basic similarities, the fundamental composition of animal and human blood is very different. Being products of bodies of the same origin, we would expect them to be far more similar than they in fact are. Where do the great differences between them come from if the blood characteristics are derived only from the body? In effect, the distinctive properties of blood must not only be considered in relation to the body in question, but they also depend on its animating core, which is the animal soul for the animal body and the spirit for the human body. In accordance with their individual natures, these animating cores then model the blood produced by the body and give it a personal touch.

This personalization of blood is essential, since the human spirit, just as the animal soul, can only act through the intermediary of the blood radiation when this corresponds to its own nature. Even though the blood radiation of those apelike animals permitted a connection for the incarnation of the first human spirits, it also remained no less adapted to the earthly activity of animal souls. The human spirit, whose potential is quite different, could not use the blood radiation the way it was without the possibilities for expressing itself in the world of matter being greatly limited. Therefore, in the beginning, the blood radiation of the apelike animals could not totally meet the needs of the human spirit. This compelled the spirit to gradually modify the blood composition so that it could become "humanized" and thus quite different from animal blood.

Something similar takes place in the course of pregnancy. As discussed in chapter 4, it is during the middle of a pregnancy that the blood of the fetus acquires a composition that allows for the incarnation of the spirit. But even if the spirit is able to connect with the body at this time, the blood and its radiation, just as the body itself, remain products of heredity and do not yet fully correspond to the particular spirit, which must still contribute characteristics of its own. This "personalizing" of the blood comes about in accordance with the law of biological adaptation. In utilizing the body in a certain way, the spirit pushes the body to adapt itself to it. Little by little, the body, as well as the blood, take on the distinctive characteristics of the individual spirit.

What Happens to the Blood after Death?

The role of the human spirit in forming the blood is much more important than the science of physiology would tell us. This becomes clear in a striking way when we examine what happens to the blood when the body dies.

Logically, if it were dependent only on the body, the blood would likewise have to "die" quickly, that is, decompose immediately upon the death of the body. The blood, however, survives up to several days after death.

To understand what happens to the blood after death, one has to understand that physical death is not the death of the spirit. During the days following death, the spirit slowly detaches itself from its cloak, the body, which it used during its sojourn on Earth. Seeing that the spirit was connected to the body through the blood, it is quite natural that it is the blood that dies last, given that it is held longer by the radiation of the spirit. When the spirit becomes totally detached from the body, the blood disappears and the blood vessels then contain no more than remnants of what was in them. Then the process of death is complete, as witnessed by the disappearance of the blood.

If the spirit remains connected to the body for several hours or even days after death, depending on the individual case, this is obviously not due to the radiation of the blood, which is now extremely weak since the body is already cold. To find out what maintains the connection, we must turn to the spirit. In effect, it may not yet be ready to leave the body, even though its body has met its end. The spirit may need a shorter or longer period of time to reorient itself, but not toward the Earth, on which it can no longer remain, but rather toward the next stage of its pilgrimage through Creation.

At this point we can take note of two aspects of Jesus's miracles of raising the dead, which occur three times in the Bible. First, these miracles took place only a few days after the deaths of the persons, never weeks later, therefore at a point in time when the spirit had not fully detached itself from the body, when the blood had not yet disappeared. If it were any later, a return to life would not have been possible. Second, the accounts of these miracles show us that Jesus's words were never directed to the body or the blood of the deceased, but rather he called out to their spirits to return into their bodies. It is only the spirit that can restore the blood's radiation, thus its power and, with it, life to the body.

Let us now take a look at the influence of the spirit on the actual process of separation from the body leading to earthly death (i.e., the process beginning before death). Here, too, the influence of the spirit is the determining factor.

Toward the end of life, with the effects of wear and tear on the physical organs, the body no longer produces as strong a radiation. Its bond with the spirit then begins to loosen. This bond, however, does not depend only on the radiation of the blood; the radiation of the spirit plays a role in this as well. According to the level of maturity of the spirit and the kind of radiation emanating from it, the bond may be broken more or less quickly and more or less easily. In ideal circumstances, the spirit has acquired sufficient wisdom in the course of its incarnation to understand that leaving its physical body means only the end of its earthly life and not the end of its existence as a spirit. It will also begin to understand that it will pursue its life on other planes, that this means progress for it, and that it can prepare for this joyfully. It will even long for this, and as it is sometimes said, the person will be "prepared."

The radiation issued by a spirit preparing to leave the earthly plane is now directed more toward the heights than toward strengthening the radiation of the blood. When the blood radiation weakens sufficiently, the spirit, whose radiation now plays hardly any role in the connection, will be released. The spirit then easily detaches from the body. A separation of this kind is described as a "natural death," and like all natural happenings, takes place without suffering. Thus the separation of the spirit from the body can occur quite quickly when the spirit has completed its time on Earth and is inwardly prepared to leave it.

In certain cases, however, the process of separation leading to death extends over weeks, and can even take months or years to complete. This happens when a spirit is afraid to leave its life on Earth, either because the separation is premature or because the dying person believes that with the death of his earthly body, it is all over, and he therefore fears death and tries to resist it by all possible means. The spirit is therefore forced to remain connected to its body. This strong desire causes it to direct its radiation toward the earthly, thereby strengthening the blood radiation and maintaining life in the body. Despite its state of deterioration, the body hangs on beyond any point possible for someone not as strongly bound to the Earth. This results in an agonizing struggle, during which the tired and worn-out body wavers between life and death, finding itself forced to keep on going, through the sheer willpower of the spirit, terrified by what it considers to be its end. The radiation bridge is then so weak that it threatens to break at any moment. We can say with good reason the life of such a person is "hanging by a thread."

Prolonging Life?

The influence of the spirit on blood radiation also explains the fact that many patients or accident victims survive despite an unfavorable prognosis, while others succumb to relatively mild conditions. With the former the strong desire to live maintains the blood radiation of the person and promotes healing, whereas in the case of the latter, by giving up too quickly, the person deprives her blood radiation of everything the spirit can provide. The will to live, though, is not always enough, because the physical body has its limitations; it was not made to last forever, as is the case with the spirit.

One would tend to expect that a person who follows an unhealthy lifestyle opposed to the physiological needs of the body to die prematurely. In such a case, the spirit has not yet matured sufficiently to leave the Earth plane and the body is already in decline. Nevertheless, a strong will to live can often be successful in making the damaged body last a little bit longer. It can hang on up to a certain point, thanks to the power the spirit can give to the blood radiation, a power that the body itself is no longer able to provide.

Seen from this point of view, life-sustaining measures for patients in a coma appear in a new light. The maintenance of heart and respiratory functions through machines, of blood pressure through drugs, and of nutrition through artificial feeding are not the only explanation for the survival of the ill or injured person. Technology is not able to give a dying person a life longer than that which has been ordained for him through the activity of his spirit.

With treatment one's life can only be extended to the normal lifespan the person would have had had his life not been threatened by an illness. However, it is impossible that technology can prolong the duration of a human life beyond the time foreseen for the incarnation of that human spirit. The treatments a person receives can only maintain the body-spirit bond and do not give life, because life does not reside in the heart or in the lungs. Being artificially stimulated these organs merely contribute to producing blood radiation, maintaining the connection with the spirit, the actual living core of the body. And it is the spirit, although not consciously in the earthly sense, that maintains life within the body.

If the spirit has fulfilled its time on Earth, nothing can hold it down on the physical plane. However, if its time has not yet come, the combined action of the spirit's radiation and the radiation of the blood can allow a person to benefit from medical treatment and thus permit the person to extend his stay on Earth. If this bridge is firm enough, the person will awaken from the coma and regain consciousness. However, if the bridge is weak, a certain connection will be maintained, but not sufficient to bind the spirit closely to the body. The body will continue to function but the spirit will be more or less unconscious in the earthly sense. This is what can happen in the case of deep comas, where the bond is so weak that simply switching off the machines leads to stopping the heart and respiratory functions, resulting in the death of the body.

Since humans cannot maintain life but can only maintain the body's ability to produce blood radiation, the dream of all those who have had their body frozen with a view toward being brought back to life at a later date, when technology and medicine will be more advanced, can never be realized. The human body is not a machine that can be plugged into an electrical outlet. Technology and drugs can only contribute to strengthening an already existing bond; they cannot develop a new one. After decades or centuries in a deep freeze, the bond no longer exists.

Let us suppose some treatment could successfully reestablish the bond. Then another insurmountable hurdle would emerge: during the intervening decades (or centuries), the spirit would have had to continue its development and would be changed. Its former body could then no longer serve it as a tool because it would no longer be suited to it. To return to Earth, such a spirit would necessarily have to go through incarnation into a new body and birth.

Sleep and the Activity of the Spirit

The influence of the spirit on the radiation of the blood can also be seen when we look at what happens during sleep.

During the day, through our activities, toxins are produced by the body that spill into the blood, changing its composition. The resulting blood radiation induces fatigue and sleep. The spirit begins to lose interest in the activity of the body; attention and concentration decrease, and there is a tendency to relax and let go. As these urges become stronger, sleep soon overtakes the tired person.

During sleep the body rests and the brain becomes inactive. But the spirit has no need of sleep. During the five or six REM (rapid eye movement) phases that are part of an ordinary sleep cycle, the spirit reaches full activity. Seen from the outside, the body is dreaming, but these dreams are, in reality, phases of special activity on the part of the spirit, in which neither the body nor the brain play a part.

These dreaming phases are indispensable for the spirit. In these moments, when it is freed from the weight of the earthly body, it is much easier to connect with its plane of origin and to gather spiritual power from the source. "To His beloved the Lord giveth in sleep," says the Bible (Psalm 127). And not only the spirit, but the body too benefits from this power because of the resulting stronger radiation.

If we systematically deprive someone of REM sleep by awakening him as soon as this phase commences (which can easily be done with the help of an EEG), and we repeat this procedure night after night, the person's state of health quickly deteriorates because the radiations of the spirit are no longer sufficient to maintain a normal bond, even though the body and the brain have had all the rest they need.

When a person lies down and his blood radiations promote sleep, the spirit can yield to this impulse and let sleep take over, or it can refuse the invitation to sleep and stay awake. The most extreme fatigue can be overcome and kept away if the spirit so wishes, because it can change the blood radiation at any moment. Danger or fear can also contribute to maintaining a state of wakefulness, not because fear stimulates the brain, but because the spirit, in reacting to it, changes the blood radiation. In this way of thinking, insomnia is due to a blood radiation that prevents the required loosening of the spirit from the body, either because something physical has had some effect on the blood composition (liver problems, lack of minerals, taking stimulants, etc.), or because the radiation of the spirit is maintaining a blood radiation unfavorable for falling sleep (obsessive thoughts, worries, fears). Sedatives can change the blood radiation to promote sleep, but they do not promote REM sleep; in fact, they shorten these restorative phases.

The spirit also influences the blood radiation upon awakening. In effect, at the end of a full night's sleep, the blood radiation is no longer the same as that which led to sleep. Thanks to the period of rest, it has again become normal. The spirit can then easily reconnect with it after awakening if it wishes to do so. If this is not its wish, it can strongly resist the gradual regaining of consciousness and may decide to continue in a state of semiconsciousness or decide to fall back to sleep and not open itself to the outside world.

If there is an abrupt awakening in the middle of the night while the connection between spirit and body is very loose, readjusting the blood radiation takes longer than a natural morning awakening. If we shake the sleeper, she does not react at first. Then she becomes aware of being shaken, but without knowing where she is or what is happening. Gradually, as the radiation changes, she regains consciousness, even though she may still be unable to move. Her level of consciousness gradually increases, and as soon as the blood radiation has sufficiently changed, she can move. From this moment on, awakening proceeds quickly because the spirit can begin to act on the blood radiation, while up to this point it was mainly the body, after being shaken, that acted on it.

If a person becomes irritable when pulled out of sleep and takes a long time to fully awaken, she may say something like, "Let me pull myself together" or "Let me come to." These responses illustrate the process accurately: the body first has to bring back the spirit by changing its blood radiation, and then the spirit has to return to the body by realigning the wavelength of its radiations with those of the body.

The Spirit, Blood Radiation, and the State of Mind

The spirit changes as a result of being confronted with the great variety of situations a person encounters throughout earthly life and having to react to them. The blood radiation is transformed as a result. These transformations do not manifest as changes of blood groups or other biological characteristics of the blood, but rather in more subtle modifications of its composition. Although very subtle, the changes can nevertheless be perceived: they are the varying expressions of our spirit, what we call our "state of mind."

When we feel peaceful and serene, that is, when our spirit is calm and content, our blood radiates in the same way. Those around us can also sense our calm state even before we translate it into words or deeds. We remain in this relaxed state until our spirit is confronted by something new. The spirit may then decide to react differently and thereby change the blood radiation. The new radiation might express anger or discontent, but whatever the emotion, it will continue until the state of the spirit changes once again.

It can happen that as a result of a lack of vigilance on our part, the blood radiation changes without our being aware of it. We suddenly wonder why we are feeling troubled after feeling so calm just a few moments ago. It is only in retracing the course of events that we are able to discover what it was that disturbed us and caused the change in the state of our spirit and hence in our blood radiation. Once the change in the blood radiation has taken place, it colors every perception of the spirit. If somebody is unhappy for whatever reason, his blood will radiate unhappiness. If he does nothing to change the state of his spirit, if he makes no effort to change and simply holds on to this state of unhappiness, his blood will continue to radiate in the same way. Such a person will be unhappy with everything because that is how his blood is radiating. The smallest things upset him, even those things that just a little while earlier did not affect him at all. He is not satisfied with anything because his spirit is surrounded by a discontent that is being maintained by his blood radiation. The spirit can then only feel and see the world through the "eyeglasses" of its dissatisfaction and not as it really is. When violent or negative feelings stir a person's spirit, then evil, thoughtless, or unjust acts can be committed without the person being aware of their impact, because rage and hatred have blinded him.

Conversely, someone who has good blood radiation sees everything in a positive light. Her entire attitude leads her to take on and experience life in this way. In addition, she will be better able to withstand problems and adversity and may even see such obstacles as a challenge to do better.

The Free Will of the Spirit

The moods that underlie our radiations may appear to control the spirit, but this is not at all the case. The spirit retains its free will at all times. While it is true that blood radiation plays a part, it only colors the perceptions of the spirit and predisposes it to feel and act in a certain way. The spirit is never forced to do anything because it is always free to make its own decisions independently.

If a person is filled with hatred, it will seem to him that hate is the only possible emotion in the situation confronting him. But in reality it is the person who has decided to color all things with hate and who has produced the corresponding blood radiation. He only has to let go of his hatred to obtain an undistorted view of reality. This will obviously require some effort on his part. He will have to overcome the difficult climate he has created for himself and, mindful of his state of mind, make an effort to change.

We know that our state of mind influences our blood. Many expressions, found in different languages, bear witness to this: A disagreement makes for "bad blood" between people. If someone is terrified his "blood runs cold." If a person is in a rage, his "blood boils." The blood is said to "turn to water" if we lose courage. There is "good blood" between friends.

When blood "boils" it no longer has a normal composition and radiation. The negative consequences of this, as we have seen, affect the spirit, but also affect the body. That certain organs become diseased because of a situation in which there is "bad blood" should not surprise us. The effects of strong emotions on the body are well known. Fear of taking an exam, for instance, can cause sweating, diarrhea, or an urge to urinate. If temporary emotions can bring about such effects, what then are the effects of hate, anger, and unhappiness when they are allowed to persist over years or for an entire lifetime?

It is true that the reverse can also occur: A diseased organ changes the composition of the blood and the ensuing disturbed radiations can influence the perceptions of the spirit. Because of a diseased body, the spirit feels sadness, irritability, or fear, because such is the coloring of the impressions mediated by the unhealthy blood. Moreover, we can see that a person changes when she falls ill and that she returns to her usual demeanor upon recovery.

The influence of illness on blood radiation, however, is still not strong enough to be able to enslave the spirit. Here too it retains its free will. If it wishes, with constant effort it can modify the blood radiation. This is made easier if the spirit can receive external help for changing its blood radiation. This can be done in a variety of ways, but the most direct way is through the food we eat—a subject we will take up in the next chapter.

~

SEVEN

Changing Blood Radiation through Food

Through the choice of foods for his nourishment man may help his body to acquire the right balance by strengthening or perhaps weakening certain radiations or by displacing the predominant ones, whether favourable or hampering in their effect, so that that radiation takes the lead which is favourable to him and thereby also normal, for only what is favourable is the normal condition!

ABD-RU-SHIN, *IN THE LIGHT OF TRUTH: THE GRAIL MESSAGE*

These days conventional treatment for most kinds of health issues consists mainly of taking prescription medication. But prescription drugs have no impact on changing the root cause of ailments, which is blood radiation. *The Grail Message* not only reveals the existence of blood radiation and its role in human life, but it also provides a clear indication of how we might go about healing ourselves by changing our blood composition and hence our blood radiation:

> Wherever a spirit is too weak to accomplish this [changing the blood composition], or wherever it is hindered in its efforts by some outside influence, such as an accident or a physical ailment, there the doctor can soon help by intervening through his knowledge!
>
> And he will be amazed at the recognition of how much depends in each case upon the right composition of the blood for earthman. No hard and fast rule must be made in these matters, for the procedure is entirely different with every person. So far only the coarsest differences have been found. There are still innumerable refinements which have not yet been recognised, and which are of far-reaching importance and influence . . .
>
> It is not through injections that *lasting* changes can be brought about, but in the natural way, through appropriate food and drink, which over a short period will vary with every individual person, yet always without one-sided limitations.[1]

Prescription medication does indeed influence blood radiation, but the effect is only short-lived. To obtain a more long-lasting effect, we have to influence the process of blood formation itself, which is controlled to a great extent by diet. Food provides the body with the nutrients that are used to form the blood, as well as the substances necessary for supporting the function of the blood-forming organs such as the spleen, bone marrow, and liver.

How we feed ourselves is not unimportant. We should of course be concerned about our diet, not only to keep a healthy weight or to have good-tasting, quality nutrition, but also to maintain a good blood radiation. It all comes down to knowing how to influence blood radiation through food, in order to provide a sound base for the spirit to further its development.

It is tempting to try to find out which foods are the most favorable for spiritual development or, alternatively, which ones are to be avoided, so as not to hinder it. Some claim that fruit has a positive influence on the spirit, and others, that meat should be avoided. However, an approach consisting of selecting certain food items is wrong, because it is too one-sided. On this Earth many different kinds of foods are eaten: standard items such as fruit, vegetables, cereals, eggs, dairy products, and meat, but also less common things like shellfish, insects, and seaweed.

The Regional Diet

Each region of the world has its own range of foods, but these represent only a small part of what nature offers in its entirety. It makes sense that if only certain foods were "spiritual," they would have to be available in every area of the globe so that no one group of people would be at a disadvantage. But apart from mother's milk, there are no universal foods. Those that one might consider as being universal really are not, because the composition of foods varies greatly from one area to the next, due to the influence of climate, sunshine, the type of soil and water, and so on. Consequently, their content of vitamins, minerals, and other constituents is different, as are their effects on the composition and radiation of the blood.

Even though the availability of foods in each zone or region is different, every area offers a full range of nutritional substances necessary for the blood. It is therefore only necessary for the people in each region to consume foods from their own soil to be able to benefit from the whole spectrum of blood radiations. No population group is at an unfair disadvantage, and nothing would be missing from the composition of their blood, as long as there are no shortages brought on by drought or any other climatic or geological upheavals.

By local foods we mean foods that are grown in the regions where we live. With respect to plant foods, these are the fruits, vegetables, and grains cultivated outdoors in one's own region. That the food is grown outdoors is quite important as it is possible to grow vegetables and fruits in greenhouses that would otherwise not survive in the open air because they have not adapted to the climate. These foods should therefore not be considered local. Of course this does not concern local plants that are grown in a greenhouse or cold frame in order to make them available for a longer period of time.

What I just said is also valid for foods of animal origin. Local milk, cheese, eggs, and meat are those produced from animals raised in the region in which one lives. The same is true for fish, which is local or not, depending on where it was caught.

The word *local* should not be seen as overly restrictive:

people can eat vegetables that they did not grow in their own gardens. Eating the products of one's region or province means eating the foods of the geographical and climatic zone in which you live, and by eating this way, you receive from foods close to all your nutritional needs.

While it is easy to see that the bulk of our diet should not consist of foods that are "foreign" to our region—meaning foods that were not produced locally—it is less obvious why we should forego foods that are regional foods but were grown somewhere else. Is there really any difference between an American pear and one that is imported from South Africa or between French wheat and the wheat grown in the United States?

Various analyses of the chemical composition of foods reveal that there are significant differences based on location.[2] The water content of wheat, for example, as well as its content of proteins, lipids, cellulose, and mineral salts, can vary by up to 100 percent depending on its provenance.[3] These differences in nutrient content from one region to the next will logically have very different effects on blood composition and radiation.

The practice of long-distance shipping of foods grown in remote locations has long been considered acceptable. For example, orange juice and bananas are eaten regularly at breakfast, although these foods do not grow in most regions in the world. The problem is not that a person is eating foreign foods that he enjoys, but that they have become a habit. In fact, instead of regularly eating local foods that strengthen the blood radiation, they are eating foods that do not have this effect, as we shall see later in this chapter. The solution here is to replace the foreign foods that are eaten on a regular basis with locally grown foods. The foods from far away will no longer be eaten every day but can still be enjoyed occasionally as a treat.

Eating locally does not mean you should never eat a food grown outside your region, only that such foods should be the exception and not the rule. Unilateral elimination of one or more foods native to your region will have an adverse effect on blood composition, because the dietary offerings of a region form a holistic group. We should never lose sight of the big picture: many different foods from one region all work together in harmony to form "good" blood.

It is quite true that the blood radiation of different populations will always show differences, given that the foods that nourish the blood originate from different soils. These differences are necessary because just as different individual temperaments require somewhat different food, so does each population group, as a function of its unique national or ethnic characteristics, require a distinctive diet. And even where nature provides a similar range of food items, neighboring populations having different distinguishing characteristics will not have exactly the same food in the same proportions in their diets.

For instance, the ranges of foods available among the European countries in the temperate zone are very similar. Nevertheless, meat consumption in some countries is much higher than in others. In one, it is eaten as is, while in others meat is prepared mainly as sausages or cold cuts. In one country there may be a preference for veal, in another, pork, while in a third, lamb. It can be observed that these kinds of culinary dividing lines coincide with linguistic borders. Not that food forms the language, but language forms ethnic groups, and the different ethnic groups require different blood radiations, thus explaining why specific groups select different foods. Nowadays, these culinary differences are not as distinct as they were in the past, because there has been a tendency to standardize our way of eating. Unfortunately—as seen in the proliferation of fast food all over the world—standardization of diets also causes a standardization of people. In this way, little by little, peoples or ethnic groups lose their distinct characteristics that contribute to their unique richness.

The Link between Locally Grown Food and Blood

There is a direct link between people and the foods they produce in their own bioregion because the physical body is constructed from materials coming from the soil where it was born. For example, when a European man goes to live in Africa, the foods he will find there are not the same as those of his homeland. They are different, adapted to the needs of the local African population. When he eats this food, his blood radiation more closely approximates that of the local population. It is then much easier for him not only to tolerate the climate of the area, but also to enter into contact with the people who live there, to swing in their rhythm, to understand them.

However, the body of the European man is not specifically made for the African diet or climate. He will become tired and worn out much sooner than if he had stayed at home, even to the point where his lifespan could be affected. The diet of a person living abroad must therefore meet two requirements: it should as much as possible remain as close to his native diet as possible, so that his body, which derived from it, receives what is meant for it; and it should also be close to the local diet, to make it easier to connect with those around him and to adjust himself to his new, chosen country.

The different dietary needs of different peoples manifest in their attitude toward foods that are not part of their usual diets. Milk, for example, is a basic part of the diet of many peoples, while others believe that it is degrading and unnatural to consume it. The same can be said of meat. Likewise, tea is the national drink in certain countries, whereas in others coffee is preferred. Wine is a drink of the West; other nationalities drink very little or none at all. In certain countries it is relatively well tolerated, while elsewhere it has negative effects, both physically and psychologically.

Food and the Seasons

The variety of foods provided by nature in different regions of the world did not happen by accident; this variety is precisely adapted to the needs of the inhabitants of specific regions, as well as to the special requirements of the different seasons.

The hot season offers the juiciest foods, including fruits and vegetables, because the need for liquids is greater in the summertime. Vegetables harvested in the autumn, such as carrots, celery, and turnips, are "dry" vegetables, corresponding with a reduced need for liquids during this season. The cold season requires the most fuel to maintain body temperature. It is also the season when cereals become available; they are rich in carbohydrates, which can be burned by the body to supply it with needed warmth. With its prolonged period of sunlight and higher temperatures, the warm season is the time when people sleep the least and remain active the longest. Wear and tear on the tissues is also greater then, and therefore, there is an increased need for protein. Spring is just when we begin to see high-protein foods being produced in abundance, the time of year when the hens start to lay eggs again, and the cows have their calves and produce milk. The availability of protein-rich foods such as eggs, meat, and milk is especially high at this time, declining in the cold season.

We have seen that the concept of the entire range of nature's offering is central to good nutrition and that all the different foods available in a given region are necessary for the elaboration of the full spectrum of blood radiation. Let us now take a look at what happens when we deviate from the principle of the totality of foods provided locally by nature, when one or more food items are left out of the diet for a prolonged period of time.

Fasting and Mono Diets

It seems curious that cutting out all food—as in fasting—has no particularly negative effects on the blood radiation in the short term. During a fast the body extracts from its tissues and reserves whatever substances are necessary for the maintenance of normal blood radiation. Of course, this possibility only exists as long as there are reserves present. When this is no longer the case, after a few days or weeks, depending on the person, the normal composition of the blood can no longer be maintained. Deficiencies develop, which can lead to serious physical symptoms and profound changes in consciousness.

If instead of fasting one follows a "mono diet," wherein only one single food is consumed—for instance, only apples, or only grapes, or only carrots—the body has, oddly enough, a harder time maintaining a normal blood composition than if it were to receive no food at all. This is because the effects of the various foods complement and balance one another. For example, taking alkaline foods compensates for the effects of acid foods, the influence of eating sweet foods is counterbalanced by salty foods, and so on.

When a mono diet is consumed, the influence of the one food item predominates, and this strongly affects the blood radiation. To compensate the body must draw all the required substances from its own tissues. This is difficult to achieve because the body not only has to extract the substances needed to restore a normal blood composition, it also has to rectify the imbalance caused by the single food item consumed to excess. If this food has a particularly marked influence, compensation will be difficult to accomplish and an imbalance in the blood radiation will follow. As well we see similar consequences when, instead of a mono diet, a number of foods are excluded, as is the case with many of the restrictive diets now in vogue. Restrictive diets, with their one-sided omission of certain foods, must be handled rather more carefully than simple diets that are only a matter of increasing or decreasing the quantity of food taken in.

An imbalance in blood radiation also results when a regularly eaten food is abruptly and totally eliminated from the daily diet. The problem for the body consists of finding a means to replace the radiation that was previously provided by this food item. Unfortunately, it is not always possible to find another food, or combination of foods, capable of producing the missing radiation. If one thinks only in terms of chemistry, it is always possible to find a combination of foods that deliver all the vitamins, proteins, fats, and so on, of the missing food. But experience has shown that this alternative solution does not suffice. Food is more than just the sum of its chemical components; each food has a distinctive nature and its own radiation.

Vegetarianism and Blood Radiation

Let's consider the example of giving up meat, which we touched on earlier in this chapter. The food value of meat is based mainly on its protein content, since meat can be very low in vitamins and minerals and, in addition, can be high in certain toxins. Chemically speaking, this protein could easily be replaced by protein from dairy products and eggs. And yet replacing meat protein by other protein-containing foods does not give the blood what meat can provide with its particular radiation. It is true that the toxins contained in animal flesh probably also play a role.

Along the same line of thinking, the meal-replacement beverages used in weight-loss diets, which purportedly supply all the substances recognized as necessary for the body in concentrated form, can certainly cover basic nutritional requirements and promote weight loss, but they are not capable of producing the same blood radiation that only real food can. Although all the proteins, vitamins, minerals, and so on, can be present in these beverages, the energy, or vibrations, of lemons, carrots, cheese, and so on that would otherwise normally be eaten are missing.

The ways in which we instinctively crave certain foods is relevant here. When we are fatigued and in need of sugar, we don't eat just any food that contains sugar. Some of us will choose raisins, others dates, and others apples. These three fruits can satisfy our body's need for sugar, but not all three are as good for restoring the disturbed blood radiation at any given time. Instinct will guide us, for example, more toward raisins than dates if the radiation provided by raisins better suits our blood than that of dates. Our instincts lead us not only toward the food that we need, but they also protect us from the foods that are harmful, through feelings of aversion or disgust.

The specific properties and radiations of foods are therefore not interchangeable. Avoiding meat brings about an imbalance in the blood radiation in the long run. It has long been observed that the main effect of withholding meat is not primarily physical but psychological and even, paradoxically, spiritual. With a meatless diet the spirit will tend to detach from the physical world, be less well-anchored on this plane, and thus cause the person to have more difficulties facing the earthly situations she is confronted with. The spirit's tenuous link can make a person feel unsure of himself, quickly overcome by stress, anxious and fearful. A lack of interest in the material realm may be accompanied by a loss of drive and joy of life. This state lasts as long as meat is avoided, but progressively changes as soon as it is reintroduced.

What has been said is only valid for someone who has given up eating meat after having eaten it regularly up to that point. It is different with tribes who have been vegetarian for centuries; their bodies have learned how to function without meat. The blood radiation is completely normal, but as a result of the effects of other foods. Certainly it will lack the "coloration" that meat would have been able to give it, and that will have consequences for the spirit. But as we have seen, these consequences are not there without reason (i.e., they have some connection to the nature of the people in question).

Proponents of vegetarianism like to cite the example of the lions who lost their aggressiveness after red meat was taken out of their feed and they were fed mainly vegetables and grain and only a small quantity of white meat. These cases are notable because they clearly illustrate how blood radiation and diet work. Despite the small quantity of white meat in their diet, the complete withdrawal of red meat strongly altered the blood radiation of the lions, to the point where they no longer displayed their normal aggressiveness toward humans. They became calm and peaceful instead. In the same situation, hunting dogs exhibited less of a tendency to fight and hunt. On the other hand, a complete withdrawal of meat did not produce the same results. On the contrary the dogs again became aggressive and started hunting, in order to find the meat their bodies needed to maintain a normal blood radiation.

Every food to which the body is accustomed, and which nature provides in any particular region, is beneficial and must form part of the diet, in the appropriate proportions and frequency. Nature, and therefore the Creator of nature, provides a complete variety of foods to nourish us. Humans can make a mistake only when they avoid certain foods because they do not conform to their own self-styled concept of what is good to eat.

Dietary Changes over Time

The time taken to change the diet is also crucial. A slow and gradual modification is more easily tolerated than an abrupt change. Sudden changes in the diet can certainly have beneficial effects on the body and the spirit, which are forced to react to the new conditions, but the benefits do not last. In the long run, deficiencies appear, along with all the problems that these entail. Even if undertaken over the period of a generation, a transition from a meat-eating to a vegetarian diet, which in itself may be desirable, is not possible without causing harm. It is much better for such a change to be undertaken gradually, over a number of generations, so that the people, by adapting and passing on the changes through hereditary transmission, can gradually develop the ability to maintain a favorable blood radiation without the need for meat.

Because it is composed of gross or dense matter, the physical body adapts to change much more slowly than the ethereal or subtle body and the spirit. However, the physical body can adapt to anything if it is given sufficient time. History has informed us that certain kings, out of fear of death from poisoning, adjusted their bodies to poisons by ingesting small but gradually increasing doses on a regular basis, so that they were finally able to tolerate quantities of poison that would have otherwise been fatal. The same thing happens with cigarettes. The first cigarettes usually make the new smoker feel sick, with coughing, headache, and nausea; but if the smoker perseveres, he finally ends up being able to stand ten, twenty, or more cigarettes a day.

The body can get used to anything; you just have to

give it time to do so. This is true both when you introduce something new into the body and when you take something away. Stopping anything abruptly, even something toxic like tobacco, is harmful because it throws the whole organism into a state of imbalance and it can then no longer maintain its normal blood radiation. The distress and the physical and mental torments that alcoholics and drug addicts undergo during detoxification bear witness to the extent of this imbalance. Although the abrupt and total withdrawal of meat or any other food considered harmful for one reason or another, as often happens with the many special diets flourishing these days, does not cause as extreme and violent a reaction as the withdrawal of a drug from an addict, the imbalance can be just as great, if less dramatic.

Protecting the Composition of the Foods We Eat

If the food provided for us by nature is necessary to a healthy blood composition, it is important—and this is essential—that they are in the state in which nature gives them to us. We content ourselves by simply saying, for example, that carrots are good for us. But we are mistaken if we believe that just any carrot is beneficial to eat. Analysis of the composition of a carrot grown in an industrial farm with chemical fertilizers and pesticides shows little resemblance to a carrot cultivated in a place where the earth has been treated with respect, using compost and natural organic fertilizers and where there is a layer of good topsoil.

A review of forty-one studies comparing the nutrient

content of organic versus conventional crops found statistically significant differences. Organic crops were of a better quality and contained many more nutrients—for example, more vitamin C, iron, magnesium, and phosphorus.[4]

Obviously, the effects of organic versus nonorganic vegetables on blood radiation will be marked. This is equally true for animal products such as meat, milk, and eggs. When farm animals (i.e., cows, chickens, and so on) are fed in a natural way and can run freely in the fresh air and sunshine, their meat, milk, and eggs have a different composition and a different taste from animals raised under confined or partly confined conditions and given special feeds designed to make them gain weight quickly. For example, one study found that the content of unsaturated fatty acids was thirty-three times higher in the meat of cows raised naturally than in that of animals raised in industrial farms.[5]

But the methods used in vegetable cultivation and animal husbandry are not the only factors that affect the quality of our food. We denature food in many ways, either by removing part of the natural nutritional content or by adding something that the food does not normally contain. In the case of denaturing, by taking something away, food loses some of its protein, mineral, or vitamin content, not with the objective of enhancing quality, but to obtain a product more profitable to produce, which keeps better, looks more attractive, and is therefore easier to sell. The three food items most affected by these denaturing measures are cereals, oils, and sugars.

Cereals contain an extraordinary wealth of nutrients in the outermost layer of the grain, in the form of trace elements, minerals, vitamins, proteins, and enzymes. Unfortunately, it is this outermost layer that is removed in the production process for making white flour, which keeps for a longer time and endows bread, pastry, cookies, and cakes with a more attractive color. We can appreciate the extent of the effects on blood radiation of whole wheat flour versus white flour once we understand that whole wheat flour contains three times more vitamin B1, six times more magnesium, thirteen times more iron, and thirty-three times more potassium.

When dietary vegetable oils are cold-pressed, they retain all of their valuable nutritional components. But if the oil is pressed under heat and undergoes solvent extraction, then it is clarified, deacidified, and treated to remove natural color and aroma, as is often done these days, then everything has been taken out except the fats. In particular essential fatty acids (omega-3 and -6), which play a central role in the immune system, are lost, and other dietary sources of these essential nutrients are rare.

There is also a huge difference between the composition of refined white sugar and that of whole sugar produced by simply evaporating the juice of sugar cane or sugar beets. Whole sugar contains proteins, minerals, and vitamins, while white sugar has nearly none of these remaining. Whole, natural sugar contains at least five times more calcium, thirty times more iron, forty-six times more phosphorus, a hundred times more magnesium, and two hundred times more potassium than refined sugar.

The absence of nutrients from these basic foods is bad enough, but the effects of these deficiencies on blood radiation and on the potential of the spirit are even more disastrous. In addition to the harmful effects of denaturing food are the harmful effects of food additives. There are thousands of substances used by the food industry as additives—coloring agents, antioxidants, preservatives, emulsifiers, gelling agents, thickeners, anticaking agents, flavor enhancers, and so on. Some of these additives are totally harmless, like red beet juice for coloring strawberry yogurt. Others are poisons or known toxins. Even though they are used in small quantities, the sum total of additives consumed annually amounts to approximately three kilograms per person, without even counting the products used in agriculture (insecticides, herbicides, antifungal agents, and so on) and the drugs given to raise animals, which are still partially present in the food we consume.

Who can say exactly what effects all these chemicals have on blood radiation, not just singly, but when combined, as is so frequently the case? Most of them are unknown to any natural diet that has ever been seen on this planet—just like the many medications, sleeping pills, tranquilizers, painkillers, and so on, that are consumed in large quantities these days.

To give the body its best chance to form healthy blood with a beneficial radiation, one should, if at all possible, eat only organically grown foods, unrefined, and free from additives. Eating a well-balanced, locally produced, organic diet is the best way to give one's spirit all the basic blood radiations it needs. A good place to start is by analyzing one's dietary patterns and making appropriate adjustments where necessary.

Establishing a Standard Menu That Supports the Blood

Let us now consider the subject of the specific treatment of the blood through diet. *The Grail Message* says there are no hard and fast rules concerning diet, as requirements are different for any given person. Therefore the first step in fashioning a diet that contributes to optimal blood radiation involves examining what one eats on a daily basis. To do this you must establish a standard menu.

Nobody eats the same things every day or in the same way. Most often meals vary in their ingredients from one day to the next. Despite this apparent diversity, there are certain constants that appear on a regular basis. This makes it possible to establish a standard menu, which is to say a menu that is representative of the kind of food a person customarily eats on any given day. It is a good idea to write this down, as the distinguishing characteristics of one's diet will appear more clearly this way. Note all food and beverages you eat and drink

- upon rising,
- at breakfast,
- as a midmorning snack,
- at lunch (don't overlook the bread that inevitably accompanies this meal or the dessert and coffee that come at its end),
- for an afternoon snack,
- at dinner, and
- as a late evening snack or meal.

For some it will be necessary to add everything that is eaten between meals and snack breaks (i.e., various candies, cookies, sweets, chips, etc.).

It is clear that the two main meals, generally those at noon and in the evening, are not identical and can even appear to be quite different. In reality they can always be broken down into two or three principal variants. And so in a meal consisting of a protein, a starch, and a vegetable, the fact that the protein comes in the form of veal, beef, or chicken does not fundamentally change the meal composition. It is a meat instead of another protein food like cheese or eggs. Having said this it is still necessary to know whether the meat consumed was red or white meat, whether it was grilled or in the form of processed meat or sausages.

In the example of the menu provided below, the different variations of the same meal are separated by an "or." You should avoid going too deep into the details, as they are not necessary. For example, it's enough to say "cooked" or "raw" vegetables. On the other hand, there is not enough detail in just saying a drink or dessert. More specific questions can be asked later when one wants to get a more extensive look at a particular part of the diet.

A person may entirely neglect to mention a food out of simple forgetfulness—eggs for example. It is therefore a good idea to review the different food groups with an eye toward which foods or food groups may have been overlooked.

We should also take note of the way dishes are cooked or prepared, which can introduce fats that do not appear in the list of foods. For example, it is important to ascertain whether you are cooking with oil (note the kind of oil) or butter, if the meat is grilled or served with a sauce, if the sauce is light or high in fat. It is also a good idea to ask how much butter is put on a piece of bread, and so on.

EXAMPLE OF A STANDARD MENU

6:30 a.m.		1 large glass of water with a slice of lemon
7:00 a.m.		cold cereal + milk + fresh fruits + black tea
	or	whole wheat bread + 1 plain yogurt + 1 cup orange juice
10:00 a.m.		1 granola bar + 1 herb tea without sugar
	or	1 fruit + water
12:00 noon		1 grilled meat + 1 starch + 1 vegetable or crudités + 1 fresh fruit + water + 1 herb tea without sugar
	or	grilled fish + potatoes + crudités + fresh fruit + water
4:00 p.m.		4 or 5 whole grain cookies + 1 tea without sugar
	or	1 fresh fruit + 1 tea without sugar
	or	1 granola bar + 1 tea without sugar
7:00 p.m.		2 egg omelet + whole grain bread + green salad + water
	or	homemade vegetable soup + whole grain croutons + Swiss cheese + water
9:00 p.m.		1 glass of milk
	or	1 plain yogurt

Analyzing the Standard Menu

Once the standard menu has been established, you'll have a good sense of your dietary pattern. It is now a matter of pulling useful information from it by asking some specific questions so that the menu's distinguishing characteristics can be grasped. This makes it possible to highlight any defects in the diet and thereby generally reorient toward corrections that are called for in order to alter the composition, and therefore the radiation, of the blood.

What Foods Are Overrepresented? Some foods appear in several meals a day and therefore play a substantial role in the person's diet, for example, when someone eats meat at two meals or cookies as snacks twice a day as well as a dessert after a meal. Sometimes a food is only present at one meal a day, but it is consumed in much greater quantities than the other foods, for example, a meal that exclusively consists of pasta or deli meats or, as a snack, chocolate. The overgenerous ingestion of one food over others should draw our attention to the disproportionate influence it can have on blood composition in comparison to other foods.

What Foods Are Underrepresented? By examining the standard menu, we can discover what kind of food is consumed regularly but in very small quantities or in normal quantities but is only eaten now and then. In both cases the food is underrepresented. An example would be when a portion of grain is eaten every day but in very small quantities or when a normal portion of raw vegetables is consumed but only once every fifteen days. The reduced amount of a group of foods indicates a risk of a deficiency in nutrients that can only reach the blood in far too small a quantity.

What Foods Are Not Represented? Some people never eat certain foods, and for this reason they go unnoticed when drawing up the standard diet. If we are not paying attention, these foods can escape our notice because they are not written down in the menu. Once the standard menu has been established, it is necessary to go over all the food groups—grains, fruits, vegetables, dairy products, meat and beans, and oils—to make sure that the menu is not missing anything. When a food group is not represented in a person's diet, this should be noted, as this absence can deny the blood certain nutrients that should form part of its composition.

Food Quantity: Note whether the amount of food consumed is normal or falls greatly above or below the average. Some people can eat very well from the perspective of food quality but in insufficient portions. They are therefore underfed and will suffer deficiencies. The consequence of this is that the blood will lack all the nutrients it needs to develop strong radiation. Others may eat healthy from the standpoint of quality but in such large quantities that they are overfed. Even when the foods you are putting in your body are healthy, if you eat too much, they will overload the body with toxins, which will have an adverse effect on blood composition.

Whole or Refined? Note whether the flour, pasta, rice, sugar, and so forth is whole or refined. As well note what kind of oil is used; is it cold-pressed? First pressing? The answers will determine any deficiencies in nutrients the body should be supplying to the blood.

Organic? Organic fruits, vegetables, and grains are very rich in nutrients. Foods grown with chemical fertilizers, as in conventional industrial agriculture, are not, and because these foods are poor in nutrients, the composition of the blood of those who eat them will be deficient. In the same vein, do the foods contain a lot of additives? These too present a risk of harmful changes to the blood composition, a risk that does not exist with natural foods.

Cooked or Raw? Many people have a diet that almost exclusively consists of cooked foods, and as a result they have certain vitamin deficiencies, as vitamins are destroyed by high temperatures. Verify whether there are any raw foods in the diet, and in sufficient portions and on a regular basis.

Locally Grown and Seasonal? Does the diet consist of a lot of food that comes from great distances or is it mainly locally grown? As noted earlier foods that have been shipped great distances do not always have enough nutrients necessary for good blood radiation. Similarly, are the fruits and vegetables in the diet in season or not? If most of these foods are out of season, they will not provide the vitality that a food that is in season can confer.

Acid-Alkaline Balance: Eating predominantly acidifying foods—meat, sugar, fats, starches—is very common today. This alters the acid-alkaline balance of the body, which in turn weakens the radiation of the blood.

Correcting the Diet

Once the dietary pattern has been determined and any flaws in the way an individual eats every day have been detected, it is then possible to implement the necessary corrections. The most common dietary mistakes follow, along with their appropriate remedies.

Quantity—Too Much or Too Little: When one kind of food—meat or starch, for instance—occupies too large a place in the diet, it needs to be reduced. Simply reducing the amount of this kind of food will mitigate any adverse effects on blood radiation. This reduction can be achieved either by eating less of this food at a meal or by not eating it so frequently throughout the day. Conversely, if a certain food—raw vegetables, cooked vegetables, or meat, for instance—has too small a place in a person's diet, the amount consumed should be increased. This can be done not only by increasing the quantity of the food in question but also by eating it more often. This food would then appear every day in the composition of a meal rather than once or twice a week.

The Absence of Certain Foods: When a type of food is never eaten, it should be reintroduced into the diet, unless the person is allergic or is intolerant to that food. It is preferable to start with small quantities, then, if it is tolerated, increase the portion or frequency. The quantity consumed must eventually reach a level that allows the person to make up for the previous lack. This goal can be achieved by adding a good-sized portion of the food to a meal or by eating smaller quantities of it over the course of the day.

Overeating/Undereating: Overeating clogs the bloodstream and therefore changes the blood radiation; this can be easily corrected by reducing the quantity of food consumed. This restriction can affect all foods or only certain kinds. It should be noted that overconsumption of vegetables (cooked or raw) or fruits rarely has a harmful effect. The foods that one should eat less of are primarily those that are high in proteins, fats, or carbohydrates. In the case of undereating, the blood is deprived of a sufficient supply of nutrients, so the quantity of food should be increased, making sure that it is high-quality whole food, preferably of local origin. This increase should be gradual in order to allow the digestive tract to adapt to the additional work demanded of it.

Refined and Processed Foods: All refined foods should be replaced with whole foods. This primarily involves grains and the products made from them: bread, pasta, rice, flour, and so forth. Sugar should also be whole and unrefined, not white, and oils should be cold-pressed. To find foods that are low in additives or contain none at all, it is important to read the list of ingredients on every product you buy. A simpler method would be to only shop in markets that exclusively sell organic, additive-free products. All processed foods that are products of industrial agriculture should be eliminated and replaced with organically grown vegetables, fruits, and grains. The organic movement continues to grow, and organic produce is becoming widely available, even in some conventional supermarkets. Along the same lines, cheese, eggs, and meat from organic farms should also be chosen.

Predominantly Cooked Foods: Reintroducing raw foods into a diet that lacks them can be accomplished by adding green salads or crudités (raw carrots, celery, etc.) to meals and by eating fresh fruits between meals or for dessert. For this to cause any favorable changes to blood radiation, raw foods need to be eaten on a regular basis.

Imported (Nonlocal) and Out-of-Season Foods:
Eliminate or greatly reduce any foods, be they plant
(vegetables, beans, fruits, grains) or animal (cheese,
eggs, meat, fish), that are imported from faraway places
and choose only local products. The widely touted
benefits of eating locally have contributed to the "loca-
vore" movement. There are many stores that specialize
in the sale of regionally produced products, and farm-
ers' markets are an excellent source for locally grown,
seasonal food. Most conventional supermarkets carry
out-of-season fruits and vegetables almost year-round;
know which fruits and vegetables are in season and
only eat those.

Acid-Alkaline Balance: The most logical way to reduce
the influence of an acidic diet is to reduce the amount
of acidifying food we eat, particularly meat and sugar,
and eat more alkalizing foods such as green and colored
vegetables, potatoes, and ripe fruits. It is also helpful to
drink alkaline mineral waters.

The knowledge that there exists a key for acting on the blood
radiation by modifying the diet was revealed in *The Grail
Message*. It only remains for us to discover how to use our
awareness of the power of blood radiation to our advantage, to
optimize our potential as spiritual human beings.

The preceding are general guidelines that can help you
regulate your diet, with an eye toward its effect on the blood
composition and radiation. Note that any changes in the diet
will be determined by the changing needs of the body, as well
as the changes in blood radiation over time.

The Supportive Role of Herbs

Medicinal and even certain culinary herbs can provide enormous support to the liver and kidneys, the main organs responsible for the composition and purification of the blood. Though the subject of herbs is vast and beyond the scope of this book, suffice it to say we can use a variety of herbs to support liver and kidney function in such a way as to maintain a healthy blood radiation, in tandem with establishing a healthy and supportive diet. This form of treatment involves taking teas or infusions regularly and before meals or taking herbs in the form of tinctures or capsules. These could include herbs that help eliminate wastes that encumber the blood, including those that act on the liver (dandelion, rosemary, black radish, etc.) or herbs that act on the kidneys (cherry stems, goldenrod, birch, etc.). Even certain culinary herbs can have a salutatory effect on organ function.

Diet Alone Is Not the Answer

Some people may perhaps think that diet is the answer to everything. Such is not the case, however. Our goal with diet is not to fundamentally change the person but to help him transform himself in order to optimize his potential as a spiritual human being.

In effect, the spirit's desire to change does not in itself transform the blood radiation; the blood can still retain all the characteristics that the spirit may wish to eliminate. However, when we strengthen the blood radiation by making the conscious decision to improve the diet, we make it easier for the spirit to change, because the modified blood radiation is now more ready to support the blossoming of the spirit. Modifying the blood radiation therefore *helps* but does not directly change the spirit. On the other hand, the spirit could just as well decide not to change, despite the support provided by the new blood radiation brought about by diet. In that case, while the latter could facilitate a change on the part of the spirit, it will not happen as long as the spirit is unwilling to take advantage of the help provided.

To illustrate this point, let's consider the many research projects on nutrition that have been conducted in prisons. In one such study, in order to determine the benefits of a healthy diet on the behavior of prisoners, one group of convicts was given vitamin and mineral supplements to fulfill their daily nutritional needs, and another group received only placebos. It was then observed that those who received vitamin supplements were generally less aggressive, not as irritable, and more level-headed. They committed 37 percent fewer violent offences and 26 percent fewer offenses overall. For those receiving placebos, the rate of disciplinary incidents remained unchanged.[6]

It would be erroneous to conclude from this account that because of the vitamins, the prisoners became better men. It was still up to them—specifically, to their spirits—to decide whether to be violent or commit a crime. However—and this is an important point—the conditions under which they would make a decision would be quite different. Instead of being tormented by latent aggression, malevolence, or continual inner turmoil, they would have the benefit of a sense of calm and inner balance and, not insignificantly, much greater self-control.

This study and others like it point to one irrefutable fact:

the crime rate would probably be much lower if those who are tempted to commit crimes were better able to hear the voice of their conscience, the voice of spirit. The improved blood radiation that comes with having a healthy diet could support the efforts of their spirit instead of hindering them. Blood and spirit would be pulling in the same direction, better enabling the person to make judicious and reasonable decisions in life. In this sense blood radiation would be a valuable aid for the changes that the spirit wants to make.

Adelle Davis, in her groundbreaking book *Let's Eat Right to Keep Fit,* describes how a group of schoolchildren who had a mediocre-quality diet (too much fat, overcooked, and generally nutrition-deficient food) were given a replacement diet that was better balanced and rich in vitamins and minerals. Their teachers observed that the children were easier to handle, more alert, and learned more quickly. They were better able to concentrate and worked harder, they were happier, and cried and fought less. Those who had had difficulties improved. They were sick less often and missed school less frequently.[7]

Here too, the changes in the children due to their new blood radiation were quite evident. Since they were better able to concentrate, more attentive, and felt better, the students worked more efficiently and learned more easily. No one had become more intelligent because of the new diet, but each one could finally unfold all her abilities and potentials without being hindered, diminished, or blocked by an unsuitable blood radiation.

For the person who desires to develop spiritually, improving one's blood radiation according to the principles outlined in this book can have an enormously beneficial effect. As the author of *The Grail Message* writes:

> It is just this which will become one of the greatest and most decisive aids doctors can offer to the whole of humanity, for the effects in this respect are so manifold that, with the right application, the peoples are bound to blossom forth most splendidly in their volitions and in their capacities, because they will be able to unfold all their power, which will not urge them on to destruction, but towards peace and a grateful striving for the Light.[8]

Postscript

Having the correct blood radiation at one's disposal comes down to the spirit retaining all its capabilities intact. A strong blood radiation provides a robust bond between the spirit and the body and transmits an undistorted picture of reality, producing a strong resonance for the spirit's life experiences and facilitating its growth of consciousness.

Looking at the state of human development today, we may be tempted to say that we have come a long way. But in reality we are still a very long way from being spiritually advanced, with love, respect, justice, dignity, nobility, and beauty as our guiding life principles. It is only in following this path that the spirit can purify itself and mature and be able to return to its place of origin—the spiritual plane, or Paradise.

The proper blood radiation is a bridge to this realm, a valuable support for the spirit, but nothing more. The onus is on the spirit to use it properly.

〜

The Mystery of the Blood

Volume 3, chapter 14,
In the Light of Truth: The Grail Message

The blood! How much swings forth from this word, how rich and strong are all the impressions it is able to produce, and what a never-ending source of conjecture is contained in this one significant word!

And much knowledge, which has proved to be full of blessing for the bodies of earth-men, has evolved from these suppositions. Through troublesome investigation and devoted work gifted ones, with their keen observation and pure volition to render unselfish help to mankind, found many a *path* leading to the *real* purpose of the blood, none of which, however, is this purpose itself.

Here are further hints on the matter, with which those who carry within them the calling will be able to build up through their knowledge of the swinging Laws of God. They will then become *helpers* of mankind here on earth in the truest sense, and as a most precious reward their ways will be brightened by the grateful prayers of all those to whom their knowledge of the secrets of the blood could bring help of a nature not believed possible, and such as there has never been before.

I will immediately name the main purpose of all human blood! *It is meant to form the bridge for the activity of the spirit on earth,* i.e., in the World of Gross Matter!

This sounds so simple, and yet it holds the key to *all* knowledge about the human blood.

Hence the blood is meant to act as a bridge for the activity of the spirit, or let us say "soul" in this case so that readers will understand me better, for they are more familiar with the expression "soul".

The spirit forms the human blood so that the activity of the spirit from out of man may proceed in the proper manner.

The connection between the blood and the spirit can easily be substantiated. It need only be realised that until the spirit has entered the developing body of a child at incarnation, which takes place at a very definite stage of development in the middle of pregnancy, causing the child's first movements; that until this stage has been reached its *own* blood does not begin to circulate; while at physical death, when the spirit has left the body, the blood ceases to pulsate and to exist altogether.

Therefore the blood itself is only present during the time between the entrance and departure of the spirit, when the spirit dwells in the body. Indeed it can be noted through the lack of blood that the spirit has finally severed its connection with the earthly body, i.e., that death has occurred.

In reality it is as follows: The human blood can form itself only when the spirit enters the body, and when the spirit leaves the body the blood can no longer exist in its actual nature.

However, we will not rest content with this knowledge, but I will go further! The spirit or the "soul" contributes to the formation of the blood, but it cannot come into outward earthly activity directly through the blood. The difference between the two species is too great to permit this. The soul, of which the spirit is the core, is still far too fine in its coarsest layer to be able to accomplish this, and can become outwardly active only through the *radiation of the blood*.

The radiation of the blood is therefore in reality the actual bridge for the activity of the soul, and then only if this blood is of a very particular *composition suitable for the soul concerned*.

In future every conscientious doctor can consciously help and intervene in these matters, as soon as he has absorbed and grasped this knowledge aright. It is just this which will become one of the greatest and most decisive aids doctors can offer to the whole of humanity, for the effects in this respect are so manifold that, with the right application, the peoples are bound to blossom forth most splendidly in their volitions and in their capacities, because they will be able to unfold all their power, which will not urge them on to destruction, but towards peace and a grateful striving for the Light.

I have often pointed to the significance of the composition of the blood. When the composition changes this naturally also alters the radiation, producing therewith correspondingly alternating effects upon the person concerned as well as upon his earthly environment.

In my lecture about the significance of the generative

power I stated that the latter does not set in until the body has attained a very definite maturity. Then a drawbridge is lowered to enable the soul to sally forth into the outer world, from which it has been protected and separated up to that time. Naturally this bridge not only permits the soul to exercise an influence on the outside, but it also permits influences from outside to obtain access to the soul by the same route.

It is not until then that the individual person becomes fully responsible before the Divine Laws of Creation, a point which has also been given similar consideration in the earthly laws.

The lowering of the drawbridge, however, takes place automatically, through nothing other than a transformation in the composition of the blood, which in turn is produced by the maturing of the physical body and the urging of the soul, and which then, through the change in radiation, affords the spirit the possibility to become active upon earth.

Here I naturally do not refer to the mechanical actions and work of the physical body, but to that which actually "leads" in these things, to that which is willed, and which the brain and the body as implements then turn into earthly deeds.

In my lecture on the temperaments I likewise referred to the blood which, through its various radiations, forms the basis for the temperaments, because up to a certain point the activity of the soul is bound up with the various kinds of blood radiations.

Since, however, the maturity, state of health and age of a body contribute to the changing of the blood composition, such a constraint might prove unjust. This is balanced by the fact that the *spirit* can change this composition, which at the same time explains the secret of the saying that "the spirit forms the body."

But wherever a spirit is too weak to accomplish this, or wherever it is hindered in its efforts by some outside influence, such as an accident or a physical ailment, there the doctor can soon help by intervening through his knowledge!

And he will be amazed at the recognition of how much depends in each case upon the right composition of the blood for earthman. No hard and fast rule must be made in these matters, for the procedure is entirely different with every person. So far only the coarsest differences have been found. There are still innumerable refinements which have not yet been recognised, and which are of far-reaching importance and influence.

The establishment of the various blood groups which have now already been discovered, and which can only confirm my statements, does not yet suffice.

It is true that these discoveries are in the right direction and have already proved very beneficial in their application. However, they remain only *one* of many ways and are not *the goal itself*, which is not merely restricted to physical recovery and invigoration, but which is able to uplift man in every respect.

In my lecture "Possessed" I point out that only the blood composition of some particular person offers the possibility for the occurrence of spookish manifestations such as knocking, making noises, throwing of objects, etc. During such incidents this person must always be in close proximity, as it is from his radiations that the power to manifest is drawn.

Even these things could be quickly remedied by the

skilful intervention of a doctor who understands, and who helps by changing the composition of the blood, which also alters the radiation and thereby prevents such disagreeable possibilities.

It is the same with the so-called possessed ones, of whom there are many in spite of all doubts. The process in itself is quite simple, even if dreadfully decisive for the person concerned and for his environment, and painful to the relatives.

The composition of the blood of these persons has formed in such a manner that it offers the soul inhabiting the body only a feeble possibility, or none whatever, to manifest in full vigour towards the outer world. However, the radiation of the blood provides the opportunity to another soul, with less good or even malicious qualities, and which is perhaps already free from its body, to interfere from outside and, what is more, to control brain and body either periodically or perpetually.

Here, too, a doctor can give effective relief by changing the composition of the blood, which in turn alters the radiation, thereby cutting off alien influences and granting the opportunity for the indwelling volition to unfold its own personal powers.

As I have already mentioned, the investigators are doing very good and beneficial work in establishing the blood groups, and it is just in the application of this knowledge that their observations are bound to confirm my statements.

If a different blood group was used in the case of a blood transfusion, then the soul living in such a body would find itself prevented from fully developing its volition, would perhaps be entirely cut off from it, because with the blood of different composition the radiation also changes and is then no longer adapted to the soul. It cannot make full use of the different type of radiation or even none whatever!

To the outside world such a person would then appear handicapped in his thinking and acting, because his soul cannot work properly. It can even go so far that the soul, hindered in its capacity to work, slowly severs itself from the body and leaves it altogether, which is equivalent to physical death.

Doctors will recognise with amazement how far-reaching and comprehensive is the influence of the proper blood composition in each human body in relation to the effectiveness of the soul on earth. They will recognise which diseases and other ailments can be abolished by the right knowledge, and how the hitherto existing "secret of the blood" is solved and thus becomes the key to joyous activity in God's wonderful Creation.

It is not through injections that *lasting* changes can be brought about, but in the natural way, through appropriate food and drink, which over a short period will vary with every individual person, yet always without one-sided limitations.

From these considerations it also follows that a great number of so-called "mentally backward" children can be fundamentally helped. Give their souls the right bridge for the development of their powers, and you will see how they begin to blossom forth and work with joy upon this earth; for in reality there are no sick souls.

Unless that which hinders the soul, or better said the spirit, is forcibly brought about by a disease of the brain, it will always and only be due to the insufficient or false radiation of the blood.

Indeed, all is so wonderfully arranged in the weaving of

Creation that probably none of my readers will be surprised when I further explain that even the type of blood radiation of an expectant mother can become an additional decisive factor as to the kind of spirit to be incarnated, which must follow the Law of Attraction of Homogeneous Species; for each of the different kinds of blood radiations will prepare only for the approach and entry of a type of soul which completely corresponds with it. It is likewise understandable that the same species of soul must try and bring about similar blood compositions, because they can only become truly effective by a very definite kind of radiation, which again changes during the different periods of life.

He who wishes to grasp this hint with regard to birth correctly should at the same time become acquainted with my explanations in the lecture "The mystery of birth," because in tracing the automatic working of the Laws of Creation I must elucidate one point at one time and another point at another time, although everything forms an inseparable whole and no part of it can be described as something which exists independently, but only as a part which is closely linked with the whole; which part in its co-operation becomes ever again visible at various places as a coloured thread woven through the entire fabric in accordance with the laws.

Later on I shall elaborate more fully on all the details necessary completely to fill in the picture, which I have today given only in broad outline.

I hope that in times to come it may prove a great blessing for mankind.

A further hint is perhaps in order: It can easily be recognised that the blood cannot be solely dependent upon the body because of the difference between human blood and animal blood, which can be discerned immediately.

The basic composition of these two types of blood is so different that it must be obvious. If the body alone would form the blood then there would need to be a far greater similarity. It therefore depends on something else—in the case of the human blood it is the *spirit*. On the other hand the soul of the animal, which becomes active through the body, consists of a different species, and is not of the spiritual species which makes man a human being. Therefore the blood is also *bound* to be quite different!

Notes

Chapter Two.
What Is the Spirit?

1. Gazzaniga, "Brain and Conscious Experience"; Gazzaniga, "Brain Mechanisms and Conscious Experience."
2. Horgan, "The Forgotten Era of Brain Chips."
3. Popper and Eccles, *The Self and Its Brain.*
4. Du Chazaud, *Ces glandes qui nous gouvernent,* 27–28.
5. Métrailler and Brumagne, *La poudre de sourire,* 108.
6. Moody, *Life after Life.*
7. Stevenson, *Children Who Remember.*
8. Abd-ru-shin, *In the Light of Truth,* vol. 1, chapter 19, "Once upon a time . . . !"
9. Ibid., vol. 3, chapter 51, "Soul."

Chapter Three.
The True Purpose of Blood

1. Valéry, *Réflexions simples sur le corps,* 924.
2. Abd-ru-shin, *In the Light of Truth,* vol. 3, chapter 14, "The Mystery of the Blood."
3. Ibid.

Chapter Four.
Factors That Influence the Blood

1. Abd-ru-shin, *In the Light of Truth,* vol. 3, chapter 14, "The Mystery of the Blood."
2. Huang, et al., "Vegan Diet and Blood Lipid Profiles."
3. Estes and Kerivan, "An Archaeologic Dig."
4. Turner-McGrievy and Harris, "Key Elements of Plant-Based Diets."
5. Pilis, et al., "Health Benefits and Risk Associated with Adopting a Vegetarian Diet."
6. Woo, et al., "Vegan Diet, Subnormal Vitamin B-12 Status and Cardiovascular Health"; Kocaoglu, et al., "Cerebral Atrophy in a Vitamin B12-Deficient Infant."
7. Abd-ru-shin, *In the Light of Truth,* vol. 3, chapter 23, "The Name."
8. Ibid., vol. 2, chapter 51, "The Significance of Man's Generative Power for His Spiritual Ascent."
9. Ibid., vol. 3, chapter 35, "Possessed."
10. *Petit dictionnaire médical.*

Chapter Five.
Blood's Influence on the Spirit

1. Kathuria, "Lead Toxicity."
2. Petering, "Pharmacology and Toxicology of Heavy Metals."
3. Klaassen, *Casarett and Doull's Toxicology,* 715.
4. Hafer, *The Hidden Drug: Dietary Phosphate.*
5. Williams et al., "Induced Thiamine (Vitamin B1) Deficiency."

Chapter Seven.
Changing Blood Radiation through Food

1. Abd-ru-shin, *In the Light of Truth,* vol. 3, chapter 14, "The Mystery of the Blood."
2. Mikulic-Petkovsek et al., "A Comparison of Fruit Quality

Parameters"; Blanco-Metzler, et al., "Nutritional Characterization of Carbohydrates."

3. Balland, *Les aliments*.
4. Worthington, "Nutritional Quality of Organic versus Conventional Fruits, Vegetables, and Grains."
5. Masson, *Soignez-vous par la nature,* 109.
6. Gesch, et al., "Influence of Supplementary Vitamins, Minerals and Essential Fatty Acids on the Antisocial Behaviour of Young Adult Prisoners."
7. Davis, *Let's Eat Right*.
8. Abd-ru-shin, *In the Light of Truth,* vol. 3, chapter 14, "The Mystery of the Blood."

Bibliography

Abd-ru-shin. *In the Light of Truth: The Grail Message.* Mt. Airy, Md.: Grail Foundation Press. Information online at www.grail-message.com.

Balland, Antoine. *Les aliments.* Paris: Baillière, 1907.

Blanco-Metzler, A., J. Tovar, and M. Fernández-Piedra. "Nutritional Characterization of Carbohydrates and Proximal Composition of Cooked Tropical Roots and Tubers Produced in Costa Rica." *Archivos Latinoamericanos de Nutrición* 54, no. 3 (2004): 322–27.

Davis, Adelle. *Let's Eat Right to Keep Fit.* New York: Signet, 1988.

Du Chazaud, Jean. *Ces glandes qui nous gouvernent, ou, L'immense influence des glandes sur le comportement.* Flers, France: Éditions Équilibre Aujourd'hui, 1990.

Estes, E. H., and L. Kerivan. "An Archaeologic Dig: A Rice-Fruit Diet Reverses ECG Changes in Hypertension." *Journal of Electrocardiology* 47, no. 5 (2014): 599–607.

Gazzaniga, M. S., "Brain and Conscious Experience." *Advanced Neurology* 77 (1998): 181–92.

———. "Brain Mechanisms and Conscious Experience." *Ciba Foundation Symposium* 174 (1993): 247–57.

Gesch, C. Bernard, Sean M. Hammond, Sarah E. Hampson, Anita Eves, and Martin J. Crowder. "Influence of Supplementary Vitamins, Minerals and Essential Fatty Acids on the Antisocial

Behaviour of Young Adult Prisoners." *British Journal of Psychiatry* 181 (2002): 22–28.

Hafer, Hertha. *The Hidden Drug: Dietary Phosphate,* Jane Donlin, trans. Australia: PhosADD, 1998.

Ho, Mae-Wan, et al. *Food Futures Now.* London: The Institute of Science in Society, 2008. Available online at www.i-sis.org.uk/Food_Futures_Now.pdf.

Horgan, John. "The Forgotten Era of Brain Chips." *Scientific American* (October 2005): 66–73.

Huang, Y. W., Z. H. Jian, H. C. Chang, et al. "Vegan Diet and Blood Lipid Profiles: A Cross-Sectional Study of Pre and Postmenopausal Women." *BMC Women's Health* 14 (2014).

Kathuria, P. "Lead Toxicity." *Medscape* (Jan. 29, 2014); http://emed icine.medscape.com/article/1174752-overview (accessed 11/9/14).

Klaassen, Curtis D., *Casarett and Doull's Toxicology, The Basic Science of Poisons, Eighth Edition.* New York: McGraw-Hill, 2013.

Kocaoglu, C., F. Akin, H. Caksen, S. B. Böke, S. Arslan, and S. Aygün. "Cerebral Atrophy in a Vitamin B12-Deficient Infant of a Vegetarian Mother." *Journal of Health, Population, and Nutrition* 32, no. 2 (2014): 367–71.

Lesser, Michael. *The Brain Chemistry Diet: The Personalized Prescription for Balancing Mood, Relieving Stress, and Conquering Depression, Based on Your Personality Profile.* New York: Penguin Putnam Inc., 2002.

———. *Nutrition and Vitamin Therapy.* New York: Grove Press, 1979.

Masson, Robert. *Soignez-vous par la nature.* Paris: Albin Michel, 1977.

Métrailler, Marie, and Marie-Magdaleine Brumagne. *La poudre de sourire.* Lausanne, Switzerland: Le clin d'oeil, 1980.

Mikulic-Petkovsek, M., V. Schmitzer, A. Slatnar, F. Stampar, and R. Veberic. "A Comparison of Fruit Quality Parameters of Wild Bilberry (Vaccinium myrtillus L.) Growing at Different Locations." *Journal of the Science of Food and Agriculture,* Sept. 4, 2014.

Moody, Raymond. *Life after Life: The Investigation of a Phenomenon—Survival of Bodily Death.* New York: HarperCollins, 2001.

Petering, H. G. "Pharmacology and Toxicology of Heavy Metals." *Pharmacology & Therapeutics* 1 (1976): 131–51.

Petite dictionaire médical, Editions Masson, Paris, 1980.

Pfeiffer, Carl C. *Nutrition and Mental Illness: An Orthomolecular Approach to Balancing Body Chemistry.* Rochester, Vt.: Healing Arts Press, 1987.

Pilis, W., K. Stec, K. M. Zych, and A. Pilis. "Health Benefits and Risk Associated with Adopting a Vegetarian Diet." *Roczniki Panstwowego Zakladu Higieny* 65, no. 1 (2014): 9–14.

Popper, Karl, and John C. Eccles. *The Self and Its Brain: An Argument for Interactionism.* New York: Routledge, 1983.

Schauss, Alexander G. *Diet, Crime and Delinquency.* Berkeley, Calif.: Parker House, 1980.

Stevenson, Ian. *Children Who Remember Previous Lives: A Question of Reincarnation.* Jefferson, N.C.: McFarland and Company, 2000.

Turner-McGrievy, G., and M. Harris. "Key Elements of Plant-Based Diets Associated with Reduced Risk of Metabolic Syndrome." *Current Diabetes Reports* 14, no. 9 (2014): 524.

Valéry, Paul. *Réflexions simples sur le corps in Variété. Études Philosophiques Œuvres I, édition établie et annotée par Jean Hytier.* Paris: Gallimard, 1957.

Williams, Ray D., Harold L. Mason, Benjamin F. Smith, Russell M. Wilder. "Induced Thiamine (Vitamin B1) Deficiency and the Thiamine Requirement of Man." *Archives of Internal Medicine* 69, no. 5 (May 1942): 721–38.

Woo, K. S., T. C. Kwok, and D. S. Celermajer. "Vegan Diet, Subnormal Vitamin B-12 Status and Cardiovascular Health." *Nutrients* 6, no. 8 (2014): 3259–73.

Worthington, V. "Nutritional Quality of Organic versus Conventional Fruits, Vegetables, and Grains." *Journal of Alternative and Complementary Medicine* 7, no. 2 (2001): 161–73.

Index